FIRST PLACE BIBLE STUDY

*everyday*

# VICTORY

*for everyday*

# PEOPLE

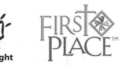

Gospel Light    FIRST PLACE™

Gospel Light is an evangelical Christian publisher dedicated to serving the local church. We believe God's vision for Gospel Light is to provide church leaders with biblical, user-friendly materials that will help them evangelize, disciple and minister to children, youth and families.

It is our prayer that this Gospel Light resource will help you discover biblical truth for your own life and help you minister to others. May God richly bless you.

For a free catalog of resources from Gospel Light, please contact your Christian supplier or contact us at 1-800-4-GOSPEL or www.gospellight.com.

**PUBLISHING STAFF**
**William T. Greig,** Publisher
**Dr. Elmer L. Towns,** Senior Consulting Publisher
**Pam Weston,** Senior Editor
**Patti Pennington Virtue,** Associate Editor
**Jeff Kempton,** Editorial Assistant
**Hilary Young,** Editorial Assistant
**Kyle Duncan,** Associate Publisher
**Bayard Taylor, M.Div.,** Senior Editor, Biblical and Theological Issues
**Dr. Gary S. Greig,** Senior Advisor, Biblical and Theological Issues
**Barbara LeVan Fisher,** Cover Designer
**Samantha A. Hsu,** Designer

ISBN 0-8307-2865-1
© 2001 First Place
All rights reserved.
Printed in the U.S.A.

## CAUTION
The information contained in this book is intended to be solely informational and educational. It is assumed that the First Place participant will consult a medical or health professional before beginning this or any other weight-loss or physical fitness program.

# CONTENTS

# FOREWORD

My first introduction to Bible study was when I joined First Place in March of 1981. I had been in church since I was a small child, but the extent of my study of the Bible had been reading my Sunday School quarterly on Saturday night. On Sunday morning, I would listen to my Sunday School teacher as she taught God's Word to me. During the worship service, I would listen to our pastor as he taught God's Word to me. Digging out the truths of the Bible for myself had frankly never entered my mind.

Perhaps you are right where I was back in 1981. If so, you are in for a blessing you never dreamed possible. As you start studying the truths of the Bible for yourself, you will see God begin to open your understanding of His Word. Bible study is one of the nine commitments of the First Place program. The First Place Bible studies are designed to be done on a daily basis. Each day's study will take approximately 15 to 20 minutes to complete, but you will be discovering the deep truths of God's Word as you work through each week's study.

There are many in-depth Bible studies on the market. The First Place Bible studies are not designed for the purpose of in-depth study. They are designed to be used in conjunction with the other eight commitments of the program to bring balance into our lives. Our desire is for each member to begin having a personal quiet time with God each day. This time alone with God would include a time of prayer, Bible reading and Bible study. Having a quiet time is a daily discipline that will bring the rich rewards of balance, something we all need.

A part of each week's study is the Bible memory verse for the week. You will find a CD at the back of this Bible study that contains all 10 of the memory verses for the study. The CD has an upbeat tempo suitable for use when exercising. The songs help you to easily memorize the verses and retain them for future reference. If you will memorize Scripture as you study, God will use His Word to transform your life.

Almost every First Place member I have talked with about the program says, "The weight loss is wonderful, but the most important thing I have received from my association with First Place is learning to study God's Word."

God bless you as you begin this exciting journey toward a balanced life. God will richly bless your efforts to give Him first place in your life. Remember Matthew 6:33: "But seek first his kingdom and his righteousness, and all these things will be given to you as well."

*Carole Lewis*
First Place National Director

# INTRODUCTION

The First Place Bible studies were developed to be used in conjunction with the First Place weight-loss program. However, the studies could also be used by anyone who desires to learn more about God's Word and His will, with the added bonus of learning more about living a healthy lifestyle.

## A Balanced Life

First Place is a Christ-centered health program, emphasizing balance in the physical, mental, emotional and spiritual areas of life. The First Place program is meant to be a daily process. As we learn to keep Christ first in our lives, we will find that He is the One who satisfies our hunger and our every need.

God's Word contains guidelines for maintaining our physical well being, equipping us mentally to make right choices, providing emotional stability to handle everyday circumstances as well as crisis situations, and growing spiritually as we deepen our relationship with Him.

## The Nine Commitments

The First Place program has nine commitments that will help you draw closer to the Lord and aid you in establishing a solid, consistent and healthy Christian life. Each commitment is a necessary and important part of the goal of First Place to help you become healthier and stronger in all areas of your life—living the abundant life He has planned for each of us. To help you achieve growth in all four areas, First Place asks members to keep these nine commitments:

1. Attendance
2. Encouragement
3. Prayer
4. Bible Reading
5. Scripture Memory Verse
6. Bible Study
7. Live-It Plan
8. Commitment Record
9. Exercise

## The Components

There are six distinct components to this Bible study to aid you in bringing balance to your life. These components include the 10-week Bible study, 6 Wellness Worksheets, 2 weeks of menu plans, the leader's discussion guide, 13 Commitment Records and the Scripture memory CD.

## The Bible Study

Each week of each 10-week Bible study is divided into five daily assignments with days six and seven set aside for reflections on the week's lesson. The following guidelines will help make your study more enjoyable and profitable:

- Set aside 15 to 20 minutes each day to complete the daily assignment. It's best not to attempt to complete a week's worth of Bible study in one day.
- Pray before each day's study and ask God to give you understanding and a teachable heart.
- Keep in mind that the ultimate goal of Bible study is not for knowledge only but also for application and a changed life.
- First Place suggests using the *New International Version* of the Bible to complete the studies.
- Don't feel anxious if you can't seem to find the *correct* answer. Many times the Word will speak differently to different people, depending upon where they are in their walk with God and the season of life they are experiencing.
- Be prepared to discuss with your fellow First Place members what you learned that week through your study.

## Wellness Worksheets

The informative and interactive Wellness Worksheets have been developed by Dr. Jodie Wilkinson at the Cooper Institute in Dallas, Texas. These worksheets are intended to help you understand and achieve balance in all four areas of your life: physical, mental, emotional and spiritual. Your leader will assign specific worksheets as At-Home Assignments throughout the 13-week session.

## Menu Plans

The two-week menu plans were developed especially for First Place by Chef Scott Wilson. Each menu is meant to simplify meal planning and include food exchanges. These meals are based on the MasterCook software that uses a database of over 6,000 food items, which was prepared using United States Department of Agriculture (USDA) publications, and information from food manufacturers.

## Leader's Discussion Guide

This discussion guide is provided to help the First Place leader guide a group through this Bible study. It provides information for the leader to prepare for each weekly group meeting.

## Commitment Records

Thirteen Commitment Records (CRs) are provided in the back of this Bible study. For your convenience these have been printed on perforated paper so that you may easily remove them from the book and carry them with you through each week as you keep your First Place commitments. Directions for filling out the CRs precede those pages.

## Scripture Memory CD

Since Scripture memory is such a vital part of the First Place program, the Scripture memory CD for this study is included in the back inside cover. The verses for this study are set to music that can be listened to as you work, play or travel. The CD can be an effective tool as you exercise since the first verse is set to music with a warm-up tempo, the next eight verses are set to workout tempo, and the music of the last verse can be used for a cooldown.

# GETTING STARTED RIGHT

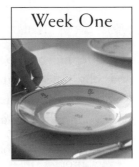

**MEMORY VERSE**

*Now what I am commanding you today
is not too difficult for you or beyond your reach.*

Deuteronomy 30:11

Congratulations! You are embarking on an exciting and spiritually reward-
ing adventure. During the coming weeks, you will have an opportunity to
see God work daily in your life. You'll discover He has given you an
opportunity to become a more powerful and disciplined Christian.

Daily prayer and Bible study are important for you to attain victory.
God provides every tool you need in your struggle for victory. You may
not win every battle. If you don't give up but continue faithfully to draw
your source of strength from God, you will eventually win the war. You
have a God who doesn't know defeat.

## DAY 1: *Unlimited Power Within Your Reach*

God understands your struggles. He also understands your potential.
As God directs your life, He commands you to take steps of obedience.
Initially, you may wonder if you can do what God commands. If self-
discipline is required, many become concerned. Is God being reasonable?
Can you do what He has asked you to do?

➤ Write out the command contained in Romans 12:1.

≫ How does this command apply to your life today?

Offering your body to God as a living sacrifice involves more than your physical body. It includes the mental, emotional and spiritual parts as well. Have you reached the point in your struggles where you are ready to offer your body to God?

≫ Check the box beside the statement that comes closest to what you are feeling.

☐ Yes, I'm ready to deal with my problems on God's terms.

☐ I think I'm ready, but I still worry about what God may ask me to do.

☐ I'm not sure I'm ready to do all I need to do about my life.

When you choose to submit to God and present your body as a living sacrifice, you obey God's command. Be assured that God will never command you to do something impossible (see Deuteronomy 30:11).

≫ In Matthew 6:33, there are two key phrases that give insights about God's commands for you. Write the two key phrases.

1.

2.

When struggling with health problems, it's easy to tell yourself things such as:

I can't get control of my weight. It's too difficult for me.

I can't exercise. I don't have the time.

I can't do the Bible study. I don't have the time.

I can't do what God wants me to do. His plans are beyond my reach.

➤ How could you use this week's memory verse to balance your negative thoughts with God's truth? What could you tell yourself?

As long as you have His power, nothing is impossible with God. God will give you confidence and victory as you work on improving your health and way of life. Nothing is too difficult when He works in you! Many times when the people of Israel were traveling through the desert, they questioned whether God could do what He promised.

➤ What is meant by the question, "Is the LORD's arm too short?" in Numbers 11:23?

➤ How does this help you know that God's power is unlimited?

When God gives you a promise, it comes true. God has unlimited power. When He promises to do something, He does it. Simply take Him at His word and expect Him to do what He says. Let God demonstrate His faithfulness today as you follow Him. Commit this week to learning the memory verse by listening to the CD or cassette and repeating the verse as you exercise, drive in your car or go about your daily activities. Keep your eyes on the prize.

Thank You, Father God, for Your promises to help me in my struggles.

Father God, give me the confidence I need to be victorious.

# DAY 2: *Mission: Possible*

When people struggle with the problems of daily life, they sometimes feel it is *Mission: Impossible*. Many feel overwhelmed by their inability to keep the nine commitments of First Place. Feelings of failure, fear and frustration compound the situation. For the Christian, the problem takes on spiritual significance and calls for spiritual answers. No matter what we say, sometimes our actions express doubt in God's ability to act in power. Even when we doubt, God doesn't react. He simply calls for a test. As He said to the people of Israel, He says to you: "You will now see whether or not what I say will come true for you" (Numbers 11:23).

➽ First Kings 8:56 tells you about the promises of God. What is the main idea found in the middle of this verse?

➽ Now that you know God has unlimited power, you know that when He promises to do something, He does it. Perhaps you have felt that you couldn't stick with a program long enough to be really successful. What may have led you to this conclusion?

➽ Write Matthew 19:26 in your own words. It contains the answer to your *Mission: Impossible* situation.

➽ Do you think this verse applies to all areas of your life? If so, how?

➤ If success depended on you, you might have reason for discouragement. The good news is that God changes everything. What is impossible with you is possible with God because of His unlimited power. According to Philippians 4:13, whose strength will give you victory over your problem?

Lord, thank You for helping me to do the impossible through Your power.

God, help me to trust You completely to help me have victory over my problems.

## DAY 3: *No Longer Alone*

If you are letting God be in control, then others cannot cause you to fail. When the temptation to omit Bible study, Scripture memory or exercise comes, call on God and ask for help. Everyone needs help. God never intended for you to fight private battles with your problems nor does He expect you to be perfect and keep all the commitments every day or week. He simply wants you to do your best. He has a better plan for you. Sometimes you may feel all alone in your fight against weight, other health problems or emotional problems. You may sometimes feel that no one else really knows or cares what you are going through.

➤ What do Galatians 5:14 and 6:2 say you are to do for others?

➤ To what is Galatians 6:2 referring when it says "the law of Christ"?

One of the commitments of the First Place program is to encourage others. Calling other members on the phone, writing a note of encouragement or saying encouraging words to others at your meetings helps you to fulfill Galatians 6:2. Jesus commanded you to "love the Lord your God with all your heart and . . . love your neighbor as yourself" (Luke 10:27). Supportive love is a key to success. God cares about every problem you face. No problem is too difficult for God.

➳ According to Jeremiah 32:17, is anything too difficult for God?
☐ Yes ☐ No Explain your answer.

➳ Rewrite this verse in your own words.

First Place goes further by leading you to think and pray about other areas of your life as well. To be truly healthy you must also consider your emotional, spiritual and mental health. Diet and exercise take care of the body; prayer, Bible study and fellowship nourish the other areas.

 Father God, help me to respond positively to the support of others in my group and to offer loving support to them.

Lord, thank You for including me in Your creation and giving me victory through Your power.

## DAY 4: *Help When You Fall*

God works through people. His Holy Spirit works within us as individuals. He also works through us collectively. When Christians have needs in their lives, God uses other Christians—His Body on Earth—to meet needs. Gods wants you to be surrounded by Christian people who will encourage you when you feel discouraged.

➤ Christians are united together in support; what does Ecclesiastes 4:9,10 say will occur?

➤ What will you do if you are alone when you fall?

Most people long for others who will care about their needs. They dream of being part of a group who will be there when they fall and help them get up once again. You became a part of a support group when you joined First Place. In addition to the support group of First Place, you have the support of the Holy Spirit.

➤ Read Romans 8:26,27 and then complete the following sentences:

1. The Spirit also _____ our infirmities.

2. The Spirit itself makes _____ for us with _____ that cannot be uttered.

3. He that _____ the hearts _____ what is the mind of the Spirit.

4. He makes _____ for the saints according to the _____.

This means that the Holy Spirit is always available to make intercession for you when you stumble and call on Him.

≫ What does the promise of John 14:16-18 mean to you in your quest for victory?

≫ According to Psalm 73:26, anyone can fail, even the strongest Christian, but what does God promise?

≫ Even without a support group, you are not alone. How do you feel about being part of a support group that encourages each member of the group? Check the statement that best reflects your feelings.

- ☐ I'm ready for a group of supportive friends; I know I can't make it alone.
- ☐ I'm interested in a supportive group, yet I'm cautious and apprehensive.
- ☐ I'm hesitant to be part of a supportive group because I'm not sure it's right for me.

≫ Explain why you checked the box you selected.

 Lord God, thank You for sending the Holy Spirit to help me when I feel alone.

Father, help me honor the commitments I made to First Place.

## DAY 5: BLESSINGS IN DISGUISE

Blessings sometimes wear disguises. Without careful inspection, you may look only on the outside and miss what lies beneath the surface.

✥ Have you ever considered problems to be a curse? Have you ever thought that it was a problem with which you were stuck?

✥ What are some of the excuses you have made or that you have heard other people make about their weight problem?

No problem in our lives looms so large that God cannot conquer it. Nothing is impossible with God. In 2 Samuel 9:1-13, Mephibosheth is invited to dinner by King David, but he's afraid to accept the invitation because he was the last descendant of Saul and Jonathan.

✥ What was Mephibosheth's handicap?

✥ What was David's reason for inviting him to dinner?

✥ Why did David want Mephibosheth to forget his past problems?

Very few people have a past as terrible as Mephibosheth's. It seemed that he would never be able to get away from the fact that he was crippled and that his grandfather had opposed the king. He was almost too terrified to accept the invitation. Have you turned down God's invitation to new life because you were afraid of your past? Look at the blessing that Mephibosheth almost missed. In a moment his past was forgiven and gloriously overcome.

Many things in the past need forgetting. We forget by refocusing our attention and energies on better things. God is always faithful to show us His footprints in every season of our lives. Once you know the story of Mephibosheth, you can never again underestimate the grace of God.

Second Samuel 9:7 is surely a message from the heart of God to you to help overcome your pains from the past: "Don't be afraid, . . . for I will surely show you kindness for the sake of [my son Jesus]."

Thank You, God, for Your great mercy to me. Thank You, God, for the good things, people and events in my past. Renew my spirit and dedication to use whatever You want from my past for whatever You want to do in my future.

## DAY 6: *Reflections*

Romans 3:23,24 tells us that all have sinned. No one sinner is any worse than any other in God's eyes. He invites all to join Him for the feast in heaven. When you accept Jesus, verse 24 becomes a gift. You are "justified freely by his grace through the redemption that came by Christ Jesus."

Since God so freely forgives you through Jesus Christ and forgets your sins and remembers them no more (see Hebrews 8:12), then you must forgive yourself for past failures. Beth Moore writes in *Praying God's Word* that "a stronghold is any argument or pretension that 'sets itself up against the knowledge of God' " (2 Corinthians 10:5). She continues, "A stronghold is anything that exalts itself in our minds, pretending to be bigger or more powerful than our God." The stronghold might be an addiction, an unforgiving spirit toward a person who has hurt you, despair over a loss, or anything that consumes so much of your emotional energy and mental energy that your abundant life is strangled.[1]

Circle areas that have given you a problem in the past because of other strongholds in your life.

*Prayer*   *Bible Study*    *Memorizing Scripture*   *Scripture Reading*   *Exercise*

Choose one of the nine commitments (as stated in the Introduction, p. 6) to concentrate on for next week. While working on all of them, add one new one each week for particular attention and prayer. When you pray, keep Scripture in mind. In her book, Beth Moore tells us that prayer and the Word are our two primary sticks of dynamite. Strapping them together and igniting them with faith in what God says He can do will help you overcome any stronghold on your life.

The key to freedom from strongholds, as Beth says, is in 2 Corinthians 10:3-5. Read this verse carefully. You can "demolish arguments and every pretension that sets itself up against the knowledge of God, and . . . take captive every thought to make it obedient to Christ" (v. 5). Using the divine weapons God has given you, pray using God's Word. The following are examples of Scripture prayers you can use today.

Father God, help me to forget my past failures and press on to the prize for which You have called me heavenward. Help me focus on pressing forward with You NOW (see Philippians 3:14).

Lord, make me like a newborn baby hungry for solid food. Help me to desire the milk of Your Word, that I may grow thereby (see 1 Peter 2:2).

Lord, help me to use Your Word as a weapon against the temptations of the flesh because Your Word is quick and powerful and sharper than any two-edged sword. Your Word pierces me even to my soul. Your Word is a discerner of the thoughts and intents of the heart (see Hebrews 4:12).

## DAY 7: *Reflections*

This week's study has focused on the limitless power of God who picks you up when you fall, gives you blessings untold and sends the Holy Spirit as comforter and friend. You have been encouraged to let God use His unlimited power to give you victory over every area of your life.

Another thought from Beth Moore is that you can take your thoughts captive, making them obedient to Christ, every time we choose to think Christ's thoughts about any situation or stronghold instead of

Satan's or our own. She writes that praying the Scriptures will give you an intimate communication with God. Let your mind be retrained or renewed, and think His thoughts about your situation rather than your own.[2]

    ≫ Of the changes you need to make in your life, which will you make first?


Focus on these Scripture verses in prayer as you make changes in your life.

Father, help me to be confident of this, that He who began a good work in me will carry it on to completion until the day of Christ Jesus (see Philippians 1:6).

    Lord, I confess to You all the sin involved in my life, and I thank You that You are always faithful and just to forgive me of all my sin and purify me from all unrighteousness (see 1 John 1:9).

    Father, help me to clothe myself with the Lord Jesus Christ and not to think about how to gratify the desires of the sinful nature. I desperately need Your help to do this, Father! Teach me and help me (see Romans 13:14).

    Dear Lord, I know that what You are commanding me to do is not too difficult for me or beyond my reach (see Deuteronomy 30:11).

Notes

1. Beth Moore, *Praying God's Word* (Nashville, TN: Broadman and Holman, 2000), p. 3.
2. Ibid., pp. 7, 8.

# GROUP PRAYER REQUESTS   TODAY'S DATE:_____

| NAME | REQUEST | RESULTS |
|------|---------|---------|
|  |  |  |
|  |  |  |
|  |  |  |
|  |  |  |
|  |  |  |
|  |  |  |
|  |  |  |
|  |  |  |
|  |  |  |
|  |  |  |
|  |  |  |
|  |  |  |
|  |  |  |

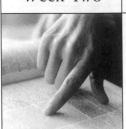

## MEMORY VERSE
*It is better not to vow than*
*to make a vow and not fulfill it.*
Ecclesiastes 5:5

What does the word "commitment" mean to you? The dictionary defines commitment as "an agreement or pledge to do something in the future . . . the state . . . of being obligated or emotionally impelled."[1]

When you joined the First Place program, you started a new venture. You were asked to make nine commitments to the program. When you read and then signed the sheet, you made a commitment. In this week's study, you'll learn more about the commitments you make and how God enables you to keep them.

## DAY 1: *Serious Business*

Today many people do not take the matter of commitment seriously. Young couples may feel they can get a divorce if a marriage doesn't work out. A young athlete may feel he or she can quit the team when it's inconvenient to practice. Commitments are easily broken. You may not be able to keep every commitment every day, but you can do your best for God.

➺ According to Ecclesiastes 5:4, what does God expect you to do when you make a promise to Him?

➽ What does this verse call a person who doesn't keep promises to God?

➽ Have you really made a serious commitment to God through the First Place program? Explain.

The best things in life require commitment. A strong marriage, a positive relationship with family and children, a solid job and excellent health are a few of the areas that demand commitment. In fact very few areas of your life don't demand commitment. You make commitments to develop in life. The Bible teaches you must weigh the cost of those commitments.

➽ Read Deuteronomy 23:21. If you are reluctant to fulfill a commitment you have made to God, what will He do? Based on this verse, do you think God would simply let you off?

➽ Why is breaking a commitment to God serious?

Have you ever broken a promise you made to someone, even if unintentionally? How did it make you feel later? God is faithful. He will never break a promise or commitment He has made to us. His commitment to you is to never leave you alone and to always give you the strength to do His will. Remember from last week that nothing is impossible with God, and He will give you the power to keep your commitments to Him.

However, because you are not perfect, keeping your commitments to First Place may not always be possible. Breaking that commitment grieves the Holy Spirit, but God is faithful and will forgive you when you don't succeed every day. Keep your commitment to Bible study and Scripture memory by listening to the CD or cassette and using the Scripture cards to memorize this week's verse.

 Dear God, help me to keep the commitments I made to First Place.

Father God, I know that You understand my desires and my weaknesses. I call upon Your strength and power to help me succeed.

# DAY 2: *God's Commitment to You*

Your nine commitments in the First Place program constitute a covenant you make with God to improve your way of life with a balance among the physical, mental, emotional and spiritual areas of your life. Whether your problem is with weight, high blood pressure, cholesterol, your heart or in your relationship with God, your commitments in the First Place program can change them. You made a commitment; that's the first step. Then God has committed Himself to help you fulfill your commitment. God not only will encourage you, He will show you the way to better health.

Have you ever wondered if there was a secret plan for weight loss that would solve all of your weight problems? Every day you are bombarded by TV and newspaper ads, and magazine articles touting some new diet program or quick weight-loss promise. Read the fine print and you'll find that most of them advocate a sensible diet and exercise. Even fad diets are careful to point out that you should consult your doctor first.

God has a better plan for you that will take care of all areas of life. The Bible tells you to look to God for help in any area of need in your life. Jeremiah 33:3 explains that principle.

➤ What does God ask you to do?

≫ And what will He do?

God's plans are described as "great and unsearchable." God's plans contain His wisdom, His perspective, His insights into who we are as people. His plans for your life will exceed any you could have developed alone.

≫ What is God's promise in John 15:7?

≫ How does this apply to your First Place commitments?

When you turn to God for answers in life, He begins to guide you. When you call on Him and seek Him, He can work in your life more readily.

Psalm 32:8 describes four things God promises to do in our lives when we seek His guidance and direction.

God will _____ you.

God will _____ you.

God will _____ you.

God will _____ you.

God is committed to helping you keep the commitments you have made to Him. He keeps watch over you and promises to teach and instruct you in all things. This applies to your endeavors toward weight loss and good health.

➤ Were you reading and studying the Bible on a regular basis before you began your First Place studies?  ☐ Yes  ☐ No

➤ If you did not have a regular study plan, what sort of adjustment in your schedule have you needed to make to study the Bible daily?

Thank God for giving you the privilege of reading and studying the Bible. Thank God that He will use what you read to give you strength and guidance in your life. Thank God that the Holy Spirit living in you will remind you of the truths in the Bible that you have learned.

Lord, teach me, counsel me and keep watch over me as I strive to keep my commitments to First Place.

God, I thank You for Your promises and faithfulness in keeping watch over me in all things.

# DAY 3: *Strength for This Day*

You can become so serious about your covenants and commitments that you may begin to worry. *How will I ever be able to do this?* you ask yourself. God understands your limitations. He has given you specific guidelines in the Bible about dealing with matters that concern you.

One of the commitments is Scripture memory. By hiding God's Word in your heart, you will have strength for each day.

➤ Consider Psalm 119:11. What happens when we hide God's Word in our hearts?

➤ Look up the following verses that will help you resist temptation;
then write each verse in your own words.

Romans 6:14

2 Corinthians 5:17

James 1:12

God's Word will give you strength to face each day no matter what
may happen. He knows the challenges you will face and will give you the
strength you need. Deuteronomy 33:25 states, "Your strength will equal
your days." Most people wish God would give them all the strength they
will ever need and do so right now. God knows best and gives you
strength as you need it.

➤ Write Matthew 6:34 in your own words.

➤ What do you think Jesus meant when He said, "Each day has enough
trouble of its own"?

God has given us a light that we can shine in the darkness that often covers our lives.

➣ According to Psalm 119:105, what role should God's Word play in your life?

He will give you His light for the path you need to take today. You cannot look down the road and see every step you will need to take in your journey to lose weight. You must look to Him with faith for each day. Jesus will give you all you need today. Tomorrow He will do the same thing again. With God all things are possible!

Father God, help me to hide Your Word in my heart so that I may resist temptation.

Lord, thank You for giving me the Bible full of Your promises and love for me.

## DAY 4: *Anchored by Obedience*

You have learned that God has a strategy for helping you to face temptation. His strategy in part involves His promises found in the Bible and obedience on your part. What if a situation develops in which you go blank and can't draw on God's resources? Don't worry. God has a plan. When you are in the midst of temptation, God promises to help you remember His promises.

➣ According to John 14:26, what will God do for you in the midst of temptation?

The First Place program includes daily Bible studies in order for you to discover truths God can use in your life. His will for your life will be revealed. Often, the truth you need will be found in the portion of the Bible assigned to be read that day.

God wants you to turn to Him for strength each day. A key way to discover God's direction for your life and receive His power is through the Bible.

➣ What does Joshua 1:8 say your level of intensity should be when you seek to know God's Word?

➣ Just knowing God's Word isn't enough. What else must you do?

God has promised success to those who seek to know His Word *and* obey it. Jesus told a story that illustrated the benefits that come to people who follow this plan.

➣ In Matthew 7:24,25, to whom did Jesus compare the person who reads God's Word and obeys it?

➣ What happens when the storms of life beat upon this person's life?

How would you describe the foundation of your life right now? Check the appropriate box.

☐ My foundation is solid! I'm ready if the storms come.

☐ I'm reinforcing my foundation right now. I'm making progress.

☐ My foundation is cracked! I'm just hoping no storms come my way.

Pray about your spiritual foundation. God will help you make any needed changes.

Lord God, I want to build my life on a solid rock foundation. Help me to spend time with You each day in Bible study and prayer.

Father, when the storms of life pound against me, give me the strength I need to stand firm.

## DAY 5: *Keeping Promises*

When people have valuable documents such as stock certificates, deeds or wills, they often put them in a safety deposit box in a bank vault. They want to protect these documents. The person who possesses these valuable documents can use them. In the same way, the Bible is a vault filled with God's precious promises. When we know those promises and understand how they apply to our lives, we can use them.

Second Peter 1:4 describes God's promises with two keywords.

➤ How are God's promises "great" to you?

➤ How are God's promises "precious" to you?

In this Scripture passage, God tells you that as you learn His great and precious promises found in the Bible, you can "participate in the divine nature."

➤ How do God's promises help you "participate in the divine nature"?

When you know God's promises in the Bible, you know God's thoughts, His perspective, His wisdom. You know what God wants and discover what He has promised to do. When you read the Bible, you know things you could never have known about God if He had not chosen to tell you. What a privilege you have. As you read the Bible, God tells you His secrets!

➤ Read the following verses and explain how each promise will help you.

Psalm 31:24




Psalm 37:24




God is faithful to keep His promises.

Lord God, help me to clothe myself with the Lord Jesus Christ and be filled with the knowledge of His Word.

Thank You, God, for Your promises to me. Help me to keep the commitments I made to You and First Place.


# DAY 6: *Reflections*

One emphasis this week has been to hide God's Word in your heart by memorizing Scripture. You have read many verses that will encourage, help and guide you every day. After you have memorized the Scripture verses, turn them into prayers that you offer each day as you prepare to face the things that will come into your life that day.

You have learned that nothing is bigger or more powerful than God. You can trust His words and His promises. His words in the Bible are weapons with which you can wage spiritual warfare against the power of Satan. God is more powerful than Satan.

God tells you to hide His Word in your heart because hiding requires intentional action. To hide something, you must first hold it and then place it somewhere. Hiding is a two-step process. Memorizing Scripture verses is one way to hide the Word in your heart. The verses become yours when you can say them without looking them up. They will give you courage to stand up for your beliefs, the power to fight temptation and comfort in times of need.

Beth Moore writes that when she prays the Scriptures, she finds herself in "intimate communication with God." Her mind is retrained, or renewed, to think His thoughts about her situation rather than her own thoughts.[2]

Remember that praying by using Scripture makes the verse more personal. The more Scripture you commit to memory, the more Scriptures you will have to use when you pray.

The following are more examples of how to use Scripture as you pray:

Father God, according to Your Word, I was once in darkness, but now I am light in the Lord. Help me to live as a child of light (see Ephesians 5:8).

Lord, I celebrate that You will soon crush Satan under Your feet. The grace of our Lord Jesus is with me! (see Romans 16:20).

Lord, I am seeking You, and You will answer me; You will deliver me from all my fears (see Psalm 34:4).

# DAY 7: REFLECTIONS

The Bible study this week emphasized how God gives you courage, power and comfort through His Word. Memorizing Scripture and making it your own gives you what you need to resist the temptations that will come as you try to lose weight and improve your health.

Remember that the weapons with which you fight are not the weapons of the world. Second Corinthians 10:3-5 describes these weapons and the power behind them. Grab hold of the divine power God provides through Scripture and prayer. Nothing will give you more courage, comfort or power in your own life.

The principle "Use it or lose it" holds true in many things in life, including spiritual truths. God has committed Himself to guide you in your life, providing the power you need to live and please Him. The Bible has all the truth you need to avoid sin and do what is right. Until you discover what the Bible says, God cannot use the Bible as a tool in your life.

Focus on these verses in prayer as you make changes in your life.

Father God, help me to put on Your full armor so that I can take my stand against the devil's schemes (see Ephesians 6:11).

Lord God, Your divine power has given me everything I need for life and godliness through my knowledge of You who called me by Your own glory and goodness (see 2 Peter 1:3).

Lord, help me to remember that it is better not to make a vow than to make a vow and not fulfill it. Please help me to realize that the power to be victorious does not come from my ability to make and keep a vow out of pure determination (see Ecclesiastes 5:5).

Notes
1. *Merriam-Webster's Collegiate Dictionary*, 10<sup>th</sup> ed., s.v. "commitment."
2. Beth Moore, *Praying God's Word* (Nashville, TN: Broadman and Holman, 2000), p. 8.

# GROUP PRAYER REQUESTS  TODAY'S DATE:_____

| NAME | REQUEST | RESULTS |
|------|---------|---------|
|      |         |         |
|      |         |         |
|      |         |         |
|      |         |         |
|      |         |         |
|      |         |         |
|      |         |         |
|      |         |         |
|      |         |         |
|      |         |         |
|      |         |         |
|      |         |         |
|      |         |         |

# THE REAL ENEMY

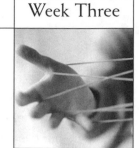

## MEMORY VERSE

*Be self-controlled and alert. Your enemy the devil*
*prowls around like a roaring lion*
*looking for someone to devour.*
1 Peter 5:8

You cannot win a war if you don't understand you are in a war. You cannot conquer your enemy if you don't recognize your enemy. Christians are in a spiritual war fighting a spiritual enemy. God gives you the strategic advantage. He provides the weapons, tactics and strategy for success. However, it is up to you to use what God provides. In this week's study, you'll learn about your real enemy. What you learn will help you win the battle when your enemy attacks.

## DAY 1: *An Enemy and a Battle*

Christians wage spiritual battles in a physical world. In his popular book *This Present Darkness*, Frank Peretti tells a fictional story on two levels simultaneously. The intriguing physical-realm story unfolds, but Peretti adds a twist: He allows the reader to see the spiritual activity taking place that influences everyday events. As the human characters interact in the physical realm, angels and demons bicker and battle in the spiritual realm. The spiritual-realm story becomes as real as the physical-realm story.[1]

Christians sometimes fail to understand the spiritual dimension of the physical, mental and emotional problems they face. You can approach your problems as strictly belonging to the area represented: physical battles are caused by physical circumstances and emotional problems are caused by emotional weakness. However, a spiritual dimension can be found in every problem you face whether it be with weight loss, in relationships with family, health problems or in your relationship with God.

The Bible teaches that a spiritual battle is raging around you.

> From Ephesians 6:12, list the four groups against which you battle.
>   1.
>   2.
>   3.
>   4.

What a formidable battle you face. Behind the scenes, the leader of this spiritual army plots strategy to destroy your life. You are not alone in the battle. Your enemy looks for anyone he can devour. This means your friends, family and members of your group face the same enemy in their lives. You can learn more about your enemy from this week's memory verse. Read 1 Peter 5:8 aloud.

> Who is your enemy?

> To what is your enemy compared?

> What does your enemy want to do to you?

> What must you do to prepare for your enemy's attack?

On one occasion, the religious reformer Martin Luther was asked, "How do you overcome the devil?" Luther replied, "When he comes knocking upon the door of my heart and asks, 'Who lives here?' the dear Lord Jesus goes to the door and says, 'Martin Luther used to live here, but he has moved out. Now I live here.' The devil, seeing the nail prints in the hands, and the pierced side, takes flight immediately."

Submit your life fully to Jesus Christ. Ask Him to be the influence in your life that will resist the devil and cause the devil to flee in fear. Keep your commitment to Bible study and Scripture memory by listening to your CD or cassette and using the Scripture memory cards to memorize this week's verse.

Father God, come into my heart and reside in me. Fill my life with Your love and protection so that the devil must flee in fear when he tries to enter.

Thank You, Lord, for Your power to defeat the roaring lion of Satan and give me confidence in spiritual victory.

## DAY 2: *Much to Lose*

Satan wants to devour your life. He knows what he wants; his goal is clear. He will use any means available to accomplish his objective. If he can use any problem, he will. Any area of your life can become a tool for Satan to use against you. Once you understand this fact, you can take steps to insure that Satan has less to work with in your life.

➻ Has any area in your life become a tool that Satan could use to harm you (for example: resentment or anger toward someone who has hurt you)? If so, briefly describe it.

➻ How can you prevent Satan from devouring you and causing you harm?

Your enemy wants to devour your life. He even wants to destroy the good things in your life. In the process, he hopes to hinder God's work in your life and hinder your joy in life.

➤ Read 2 Corinthians 11:14. How does Satan disguise himself in order to fool you?

➤ Who is the only true light?

➤ How has Satan disguised himself and used his wiles in an attempt to devour you and cause you to question God's power in your life (for example, stress on the job)?

➤ How can you defeat Satan?

➤ Has anything in your life allowed Satan to devour your confidence and self-esteem? If so, how can you defeat it?

➤ Have your actions toward others provided Satan an opportunity to undermine your testimony to others about Christ? If so, how can you defeat Satan?

If you are uncertain how to defeat Satan in these areas, ask your Christian friends to give you prayer support. Your First Place group will pray for you, even if you don't go into detail about your prayer need.

Jesus recognized the need for a little help from friends. In Mark 2:1-5 is the story of a man who was paralyzed. He desperately needed to get to Jesus and find help. His persistent friends helped.

➤ Jesus saw something in the man's friends. What did Jesus see and what impact did it have?




The man's friends refused to stop until their paralyzed friend experienced Jesus' fullest work in his life. For many people, problems can become emotionally paralyzing. They have failed so often in attempts to solve their problems that they find it difficult to bring the problem to God alone. Like the paralyzed man, everyone at some point needs help bringing needs to Jesus.

The Old Testament prophet Joel spoke words of hope from God to people whose lives had been devastated by swarms of locusts.

➤ In Joel 2:25, what did God tell the people?




You can take comfort in this truth: What you have lost to Satan, God can restore.

Lord, thank You for restoring joy and happiness in my life through Your love. God, thank You for providing Christian friends who pray and offer me support in time of need.

# DAY 3: *Spiritual Strongholds*

In military terms, a stronghold is an occupied position that provides both defensive and offensive benefits. The defensive benefit is that the stronghold is positioned in such a way that it can easily be held and defended. The offensive benefit is that the stronghold provides a strategic position from which to launch attacks on an unsuspecting foe.

The Bible speaks of spiritual strongholds. Such strongholds are good or bad, depending on who occupies them.

➾ How did David describe the Lord in Psalm 27:1,2?

Obviously David experienced the positive benefits of having a stronghold in life occupied by God. Second Corinthians 10:4-6 describes a negative stronghold—one occupied by Satan and his forces.

➾ How are you to fight Satan according to verse 4?

➾ How can arguments and pretension that set themselves up against the knowledge of God become a stronghold?

➾ How can negative thoughts become a stronghold? What must be done with them?

➾ How can acts of disobedience become a stronghold? What must be done?

Satan's primary stronghold in the lives of Christians is their thoughts. Since thoughts can lead to actions, evil thoughts can lead to evil actions. Ultimately, you must take personal responsibility for confronting the spiritual strongholds in your life. Friends can help. The time comes, however, when you must deal personally with Satan—in God's power.

James 4:7 reveals two actions to take in dealing with Satan and his stronghold in your life.

⟫ How can you submit yourself to God?

⟫ What have you learned that can help you resist Satan with confidence?

⟫ What happens when you resist Satan?

God has given you full life in Jesus Christ. He has set you free!

Father God, thank you for my life so full and free. Help me to serve You faithfully.

Lord, Your promises of help in time of need give me hope for the future.

## DAY 4: *God's Stronghold or Satan's Stronghold*

The Bible says someone will occupy the stronghold in your life—God or Satan. If you do allow God full access to your life, Satan will seek to exert any influence he can over you. Initially, Satan will settle for a foothold, some part of your life in which he can exert control. In time, Satan hopes that tiny foothold can become a stronghold. God has built a strong wall of faith around you. If any little part begins to crumble, Satan pounces on it and begins to pick away at it until he can get his hand through. He'll continue to work until he can get inside the wall and begin to weaken it from inside. All Christians need to be on guard against Satan, who prowls around just looking for the weak spots in their lives.

The more you learn about Satan and his strategy, the more effectively you can battle him.

➣ In John 10:10, how does Jesus describe Satan and what he seeks to do in your life?

➣ Think about various situations in your life. In what ways has Satan attempted to use any of them to steal, kill and destroy your life?

Satan will use any foothold in your life to harm you. Jesus, however, can use any foothold in your life to do incredibly positive things.

➣ What does John 10:10 say Jesus wants to accomplish in our lives?

➣ What do you think Jesus meant by the phrase "have life . . . to the full"?

≫ According to 1 John 4:4, who is the one who is in you and greater than the one in the world?

Paul assures Christians with a great promise for the fight against Satan and the lures of the world.

≫ Write the promise of 2 Timothy 4:18 in your own words.

≫ In Romans 7:24, how did Paul refer to himself?

≫ What did he want someone to do for him? How did he describe his body?

When you reach a point of despair in your life, you position yourself for God to work in you. Turn your problem over to God. Trust Him to break the stronghold.

 Lord God, help me to spend time in Your Word so that I can resist the wiles of Satan as he seeks to devour me.

Father, thank You for giving me a full life and setting me free from the clutches of Satan.

# DAY 5: *Ready for Action*

Many things, including poor eating habits and lack of exercise can become a stronghold in your life. Satan can use this foothold, develop it and strengthen it until it becomes a negative spiritual stronghold. You must take decisive action to remove Satan's destructive influence in your life. Satan takes indecision and turns it to his benefit.

The initial step in dislodging Satan's stronghold is to come to the place where you will no longer tolerate his influence. At that point, you commit yourself to taking whatever action is necessary to remove him.

Sometimes your own faith is weak. Believing God will actually help you is sometimes difficult. In that situation, it's possible for you to benefit from the faith of others. Even Paul struggled with sin in his life.

➤ According to Romans 7:15, how did Paul feel about the sins with which he struggled?

➤ How can Paul's statement apply to you as you battle strongholds in your life?

The frustration Paul expressed about sin certainly applies today. The good news is that no matter what the sin is, God forgives and restores the joy of salvation. David gave in to the temptation Satan set before him and committed adultery with Bathsheba. In addition, David arranged to have Bathsheba's husband put in the forefront of battle so that he could be killed. When the priest Nathan confronted David, he repented and asked God's forgiveness.

➤ Read Psalm 51:1-4,10-12,17. Verses 1 through 4 are David's confession and plea. What was his plea?

≫ Against whom did David sin?

≫ What does David ask of God in verses 10 through 12?

≫ According to verse 17, what are the sacrifices that please God?

How comforting to know that Christians have a compassionate and loving God who forgives His children in repentance. When you look at men and women in the Bible, you can benefit from their faith, but before others can help you deal with spiritual problems, you must open up your life and confess just as David and so many others did. James 5:16 gives guidelines for opening up to and trusting in fellow Christians.

≫ What must you do with other believers?

≫ What benefits will you receive?

Being honest with your Christian friends about the struggles you face in your life will bring powerful prayer support to encourage you and sustain you through any struggle. Your First Place friends' prayer for you and your prayers for them give you the opportunity to keep your commitment of encouragement.

Lord God, thank You for the Christian friends You give me through the First Place program. Help me to be an encourager and helper to them.

Oh, Father God, create in me a clean heart and forgive me when my faith is weak and I give in to the power of Satan.

## DAY 6: *Reflections*

In this week's study you have learned how circumstances in life can become a stronghold and weaken your faith. Think about what a stronghold is. Beth Moore defines a stronghold as anything that exalts itself in your mind and pretends to be bigger or more powerful than God. Strongholds steal much of your focus and can cause you to feel overpowered. Moore refers to your struggle as warfare waged by the enemy with the primary battlefield being your mind.[2]

The strongest weapons against any stronghold are Scripture and prayer. Memorizing Scripture and using those verses in prayer gives you such a powerful weapon that Beth Moore compares it to two sticks of dynamite strapped together to demolish the enemy.[3]

You serve a Savior so powerful that Satan flees from His presence. When you call upon the power of God to help you overcome strongholds, you call down a weapon that renders Satan powerless in your life. Remember, God is on your side and He cares about you. He wants the best for you, and His best for you includes confessing your sin and turning away from Satan. With God's Word in your heart and mind, Satan can't even get a toehold much less a foothold in your life.

The following are examples of using Scripture to defeat your enemy. The prayers are from Beth Moore's book, *Praying God's Word.*

Who is like Your children, O God, a people saved by the Lord? You are my shield and helper and my glorious sword. Cause my enemy to cower, Lord! Trample down his high places [see Deuteronomy 33:29].

Keep me safe, O God, for in You I take refuge. I say to You, Lord, "Your are my Lord; apart from you I have no good thing" [see Psalm 16:1,2].

Lord God, I will shout for joy when You make me victorious, and I will lift up a  banner in the name of my God! Please, Lord, grant these requests [see Psalm 20:5].[4]

# DAY 7: *Reflections*

This week's Bible study emphasized how God gives you courage and power to fight the wiles of Satan. Confessing sins and seeking forgiveness daily in your prayers sets up obstacles that Satan finds difficult to climb. God gives you what you need each day to fight against evil and your own sinful nature.

So many times when sin is mentioned or discussed at length, people have a tendency to think about sins such as sexual sin, murder, slander, stealing or addictions. These are sins, but not the ones you face daily. Paul reminds you that everyone has a sinful nature. The sins you commit are usually those that involve your relationships with others, unhealthy lifestyle habits, a broken promise, resentment or anger. These must be confessed daily.

You may even believe that those are not really sins. Think about each thing mentioned; then acknowledge each as a weakness if it applies to you, and seek God's help in overcoming it. Some of the weaknesses that many face include making excuses for not exercising, eating or drinking unhealthy foods, being unkind and hurtful to someone, holding a grudge or resentment against another, not really believing that God will take care of you, making a promise to God and then making excuses for not keeping it, failing to hold your tongue and saying things you shouldn't say, not responding to the needs of others, not giving back to God a portion of what He has given you, keeping silent instead of voicing your concern or belief, or failing to use an opportunity to witness when God gives you one. No matter how strong a Christian is, seemingly little things can creep in, build up and slowly destroy your spirit.

Don't be discouraged. You have great hope in the Father. Reread the great promises of this week's study. Be strong in the Lord, and He will give you great victory. Use the weapons God provides, and defeat even Satan, the one who seeks to devour you.

Focus on the following verses in prayer as you make changes in your life:

Lord, I confess my sin to You because You have promised that if I confess my sin, You will be faithful to forgive my sin and will purify me from all unrighteousness (see 1 John 1:9).

Lord, preserve me from all evil and preserve my soul. Preserve my going out and my coming in from this time forth and forevermore (see Psalm 121:7,8).

Lord God, You are my light and my salvation; whom shall I fear? You are the strength of my life; of whom shall I be afraid? (see Psalm 27:1).

Lord, help me to be self-controlled and alert so that I might defeat Satan who prowls around like a roaring lion seeking someone to devour (see 1 Peter 5:8).

Notes

1. Frank Peretti, *This Present Darkness* (Wheaton, IL: Crossway Books, 1986).
2. Beth Moore, *Praying God's Word* (Nashville, TN: Broadman and Holman, 2000), p. 3.
3. Ibid., p. 6.
4. Ibid., pp. 313, 314, 316.

# GROUP PRAYER REQUESTS  TODAY'S DATE:_____

| NAME | REQUEST | RESULTS |
|------|---------|---------|
|      |         |         |
|      |         |         |
|      |         |         |
|      |         |         |
|      |         |         |
|      |         |         |
|      |         |         |
|      |         |         |
|      |         |         |
|      |         |         |
|      |         |         |
|      |         |         |

# OUR SPIRITUAL WEAPONS

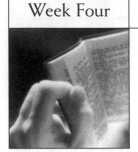

## MEMORY VERSE

*The weapons we fight with are not the weapons of the world. On the contrary, they have divine power to demolish strongholds.*

2 Corinthians 10:4

God gives you weapons to use in your spiritual battle. These powerful weapons enable you to pull down the negative spiritual strongholds in your life and defeat Satan.

God provides all you need to wage spiritual warfare. In this week's study, you'll learn more about five spiritual weapons:

1. The name of Jesus
2. The blood of Jesus
3. Your testimony for Christ
4. Your commitment to Jesus Christ
5. The Word of God and prayer

## DAY 1: *Counterattack with the Name of Jesus*

God never intended for you as a Christian to wait passively for Satan to attack. God equips you to withstand Satan's attacks. God prepares you to mount an offensive and expects you to use your spiritual weapons to attack Satan and put him on the defensive.

➤ James 4:7 explains the initial steps you must take in your counterattack against Satan. What are the two steps mentioned in this verse?

1.

2.

When you submit to God and resist Satan, you serve notice that you have shifted from defense to offense in dealing with him. When you submit to God, you yield your life to Him, acknowledging His right to rule in your life and voluntarily giving Him a position of prominence.

James 4:7,8 describes how to resist Satan. You have to resist him in every situation in your life. Satan is "the father of lies" (John 8:44), and he uses lies to discourage and distract you.

➤ As Satan looks for moments of weakness to exploit, what can you say and do to express resistance?

Times of weakness are when to put into practice what you have learned about prayer and Scripture. When you submit to God and resist the devil, you lay a foundation for your spiritual counterattack. As Satan flees, launch your full-scale attack.

➤ According to Philippians 2:9-11, what will happen when the name of Jesus is spoken?

What a beautiful, powerful picture! Even Satan one day must confess on bended knee that Jesus Christ is Lord. Don't lose heart because so many disregard Jesus' name now. In the spiritual realm, the truth is known already. Among Satan and his demons, the mention of Jesus' name makes them shudder and flee. First John 4:4 describes the truth already known in the spiritual realm.

➤ What is the truth found in 1 John 4:4 that encourages you as you fight in Jesus' name?

≫ According to James 2:19, what is the response of the demons and Satan to the name of Jesus? Why do they have this response?

≫ John 14:13 contains another promise regarding Jesus' name. What does Jesus promise to do for His children and why?

The use of Jesus' name is not a ritual for producing spiritual results. Jesus' name can't be used flippantly as part of a spiritual war game. On the contrary, use Jesus' name because God gives you authority to represent Jesus, His kingdom and His character in the world. The name of Jesus is the legal authorization that allows us to stand against the devil.

Thank You, Lord, for giving me the privilege of representing Jesus Christ in the world today.

Dear Father, help me to bring glory to Your name through the witness of my life.

# DAY 2: *The Blood of Jesus in the Ongoing Battle*

The book of Revelation reveals Satan's ultimate defeat. People new to Christianity and the Bible sometimes get confused by the passages about the blood of Jesus. Revelation 12:10,11 describes the effectiveness of Jesus' blood as our second spiritual weapon.

≫ Leviticus 17:11 describes the Old Testament system of blood sacrifice for atonement. What was the purpose of the blood sacrifice?

How does blood atonement defeat Satan?

In the Bible, blood always represents life. When the Bible speaks of the "blood of Christ," you can substitute the words "life of Christ." When the Bible speaks of Christ shedding His blood, think of Christ giving His life. The ideas are interchangeable.

In following the list, read the verses; then complete the phrase describing what Christ's blood accomplished for you.

1. Romans 5:9—I am _____ by Jesus' blood.

2. Ephesians 1:7—I have _____ through Jesus' blood.

3. Ephesians 2:13—I have been _____ to God through the blood of Christ.

4. Colossians 1:20—I am _____ to God through His blood.

5. Revelation 1:5—I have been _____ my sins by His blood.

Each day Christians fight spiritual battles, but through the blood of Christ we are promised victory. You have the spiritual weapons to defeat Satan, but he will return again to fight another battle. Satan even tempted Jesus in the wilderness, and Jesus defeated him using God's Word.

➤ In Luke 4:13, how did Satan respond when Jesus continued to resist him?

➤ What did Satan decide to wait for? How does that relate to your struggles with temptations and trials?

Although you continue to battle now, Revelation 20:10 tells us what will happen to Satan in the end. Satan is already defeated through Christ's death on the cross. His battles now are simply the last gasp of an enemy who refuses to admit defeat. Don't be deceived by this appearance of weakness. Satan's grip on those not always on guard can be strong. Stay alert, do not become weary, and don't give up. Giving up is the only way you can lose the battle. Claim the promise in Galatians 6:9.

➤ If you do not weary in doing good, what will be your reward?

Lord, give me the strength to persevere and not give up in battle against Satan.

Father God, I claim Your promises and know that You will stand beside me as I face the temptations and troubles of each day.

## DAY 3: *Your Testimony as a Christian*

The third weapon of your warfare is found in the latter part of Revelation 12:11.

⇛ What is the third weapon that we have?

⇛ What does your testimony for Jesus prove to Satan?

⇛ On what is your testimony based?

If you truly trust in the blood of Jesus to save you, your testimony will become a powerful weapon.

⇛ What is the basis of the believer's testimony as stated in 1 John 5:11,12?

⇛ According to Titus 3:5, what are the results of a right relationship with God?

Before you can experience spiritual victory, you must be sure that Jesus does live in you. Those without Christ in their lives will suffer ongoing defeat. Trusting church membership, a relationship with others, or any other sort of good work you do, you have been deceived. You become a Christian on the basis of God's mercy. When Christ died, He made it possible for everyone to become Christians. He paid the debt of sin you owed but could never pay.

≫ Romans 10:9,13 clarify the steps a person takes to become a Christian. List the three steps.

1.

2.

3.

If you have not taken these steps, now is the time. Ask God to give you His saving grace. He will because He has promised to do so. If you are unsure about the steps and what you must do, talk with your First Place leader.

Once God comes into your life, He will send the Holy Spirit to help you fight your battles with Satan. Sharing God's Word and letting others know of your salvation, gives you access to the most powerful weapons against evil that can exist. Even the unsaved can call on Jesus' name in time of crisis, but without the full knowledge of His saving grace, their efforts are weak and ineffectual.

≫ Read the following verses about the testimony of Christians; then answer the questions.

1. Acts 14:3—What happens when Christians speak boldly for the Lord?

2. 2 Timothy 1:8,9—What did Paul instruct Timothy to do and why?

3. 1 John 4:14-16—What is your reward for testifying that God sent His Son, Jesus, to be the Savior of the world?

What does the everyday testimony of your life tell others about your relationship with Jesus?

Father God, I praise Your name. Let my life be a testimony to the supreme sacrifice of Your Son, Jesus.

Lord, give me a boldness that will enable me to tell others of Your great gift. Help me to use my testimony as a weapon against Satan.

## DAY 4: *Commitment to Win the War Through Jesus*

The fourth weapon you can use to fight Satan is your total commitment to Jesus Christ. If you want to have victory over Satan, you must be totally sold out to Jesus.

In Revelation 12:11 John describes those who overcome Satan. Do you see how testimony and commitment go hand-in-hand?

According to the latter part of this verse, how strong was their commitment?

According to Matthew 16:24, what are the three steps Jesus asks you to make as one of His disciples?

1.

2.

3.

If you do these three things daily in your life, you demonstrate that you are fully committed to Jesus Christ. If, however, you have any attitudes or activities that you are unwilling to surrender to Christ's control, Satan recognizes your lack of commitment. He will then attempt to keep you in spiritual bondage.

> In Psalm 37:5,6, what is God's promise to you for committing your whole life to Him?

> What is the promise found in Proverbs 16:3?

> What is Paul's testimony of commitment in 2 Timothy 1:12?

Committing your life to Christ involves everything about your life, including your possessions, time, daily activities and your dreams and plans for the future. Without a full commitment of everything in your life, you leave a corner or a little space where Satan can poke in a finger to dig around until he gets his hand, then his head, then his body into your life.

Examine the areas of your life where you may lack total commitment, including the areas of commitment in the First Place program. Keeping all nine commitments every day every week is difficult for everyone, but the memory verse from Week One reminds you that what He asks is "not too difficult for you or beyond your reach." Commit each day to Him and let Him help you. Read 1 John 4:4. Consider now any areas of your life that have not been fully yielded to Christ's control. These might include your weight concern; stress on the job; relationships with others; or making excuses for skipping prayer, Bible study or exercise.

≫ According to Proverbs 28:13, what happens when you try to hide your sins?

≫ What will happen when you confess and renounce your sins?

 Lord God, I confess my sins to You and seek forgiveness so that my life may be a testimony of Your great love and mercy to all people.

Father, I turn my commitments over to You and ask that You lead me in Your ways each day.

## DAY 5: God's Word—The Ultimate Weapon

Your fifth weapon of warfare is described in Ephesians 6:17.

≫ How does Ephesians 6:17 describe this ultimate weapon?

≫ In 2 Timothy 2:15, you are told what to do with His Word. Complete the following:

1. In your use of the Bible, you should seek the approval of

_____.

2. In your skillful use of the Bible, you should be like a workman

_____.

3. If you were evaluated by God, you would not want to be

                    _____.

4. Your goal with the Bible is to _____ the
   word of truth.

Reading God's Word is not enough. Memorizing God's Word is the best way to insure that you are fully armed at all times. Not memorizing and trying to use God's Word is like carrying around an unloaded gun. Scripture memory gives you the ammunition you need to keep your weapon fully loaded and ready at all times.

If you want to put on the whole armor of God, you must include Scripture memory and Bible study. Not only does the study of God's Word provide you with a powerful weapon with which to defeat Satan, but it also helps you in many other ways.

➤ Read the following verses; then match them with the key phrases.

_____ Psalm 119:9      a. God's Word helps me live a pure life.

_____ Psalm 119:11    b. Don't merely read God's Word; obey it.

_____ James 1:22      c. God's Word helps me resist sin.

➤ In spiritual battles you must be constantly prepared. You must use all five spiritual weapons God has given you. List the five spiritual weapons you have learned about this week.

1.

2.

3.

4.

5.

≫ Of these five, why is memorizing and using God's Word important to you?

≫ For each spiritual weapon, write one specific action you can take to make that commitment true in your life.

1.

2.

3.

4.

5.

 Lord God, I pray for Your strength in keeping my commitments to You each day.

Oh, Father God, continue to help me to hide Your Word in my heart so that I may not sin against You.

## DAY 6: *Reflections*

This week you have learned about the spiritual weapons that are available for your battle against Satan. Each of them is important in demolishing the strongholds that come into your life. Last week two of them were compared to two sticks of dynamite. Beth Moore's book *Praying God's Word* is all about taking the two primary sticks of dynamite, prayer and God's Word, and igniting them with faith in what God says He can do.

In her book, Moore explains how the two can be so powerful. Prayer keeps you in constant communion with God, which should be the goal of a believer's life. Prayerful lives are powerful lives. However, she is quick to point out that the ultimate goal God has for you is not power but personal intimacy with Him. An intimate personal relationship with God should be the focus, not warfare. The primary strength is godliness which is achieved only through intimacy with God. For this reason God reinforces prayer as one of the weapons of warfare because His chief objective is to keep you entirely connected to Him.[1]

Prayer brings victory, but the greater victory is a closer, more intimate relationship with Him. Moore points out that the fastest way to lose your balance in warfare is to rebuke the devil more than you relate to God.[2]

When you make friends, how do you get to know them? By spending time with them of course. When you spend time with someone, you come to know them personally rather than relying on what someone else tells you about that person. The only way to get to know God personally is to communicate with Him, spend time with Him and commit your life to Him.

Use your prayer time this week to pray for the spiritual discernment to keep yourself balanced on the battlefield. The following are examples of using Scripture in prayer at times when you feel that Satan is trying to defeat you:

> Who among the gods is like You, O Lord? Who is like You—majestic in holiness, awesome in glory, working wonders? Stretch out Your right hand and deal with my enemy, O God! (see Exodus 15:11,12).
>
> Lord God, the cords of death have entangled me; the torrents of destruction are overwhelming me. The cords of the grave have coiled around me; the snares of death are confronting me. In my distress I am crying to You, my God, for help. From Your Temple hear my voice; let my cry come before You into Your ears (see Psalm 18:4-6).
>
> I trust in You, Lord, so You will rescue me. Teach me how to delight in You. Deliver me, O God (see Psalm 22:8).[3]

## DAY 7: Reflections

This week's Bible study emphasized how through His Word God gives you power to fight the wiles of Satan.

Studying and reading God's Word reveals His promises to you. In His Word you learn about His love for you and His great mercy for you as a sinner. He teaches you how to overcome the temptations of Satan. He shows you how to live your life in total commitment to Him. He shows you that He sent the Holy Spirit to guide you each day.

Beth Moore believes that she has never discovered a more powerful way to demolish strongholds in her life than praying Scripture. Although she doesn't always pray using Scripture, when it comes to warfare, this approach is the one she applies most often. By reading God's Word, you equip yourself with Scripture you can then use as a weapon against Satan.[4]

Focus on the following Scripture verses in prayer as you equip yourself to defeat your enemy:

 In my anguish I cry to You, Lord. Answer me by setting me free! You, O Lord, are with me; I will not be afraid. You are my helper. I will look in triumph at my enemies (see Psalm 118:5-7).

Father, I pray that You will see that no weapon forged against me will prevail. Enable me to refute the tongue of my accuser. Thank You for giving this as my heritage as Your servant, O Lord (see Isaiah 54:17).

Father God, I thank You that because I am in Christ, Satan, the prince of this world, has no hold on me (see John 14:30).

Lord, though I live in the world, I do not wage war as the world does. The weapons I fight with are not the weapons of the world. On the contrary, they have divine power to demolish strongholds (see 2 Corinthians 10:4).

**Notes**
1. Beth Moore, *Praying God's Word* (Nashville, TN: Broadman and Holman, 2000), pp. 6, 7.
2. Ibid., p. 7.
3. Ibid., pp. 312, 314-315, 317.
4. Ibid., p. 8.

# GROUP PRAYER REQUESTS   TODAY'S DATE:_____

| NAME | REQUEST | RESULTS |
|------|---------|---------|
|      |         |         |
|      |         |         |
|      |         |         |
|      |         |         |
|      |         |         |
|      |         |         |
|      |         |         |
|      |         |         |
|      |         |         |
|      |         |         |
|      |         |         |
|      |         |         |
|      |         |         |
|      |         |         |

# PRAYER: OUR BATTLEGROUND

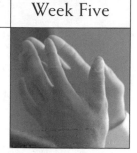

### MEMORY VERSE
*Call to me and I will answer you and tell you*
*great and unsearchable things you do not know.*
Jeremiah 33:3

Prayer is not just one of the spiritual weapons you use to attack the enemy. Prayer *is* the battleground.

Using the five spiritual weapons you studied last week will produce an effective prayer life. You will be ready to step onto the battlefield and claim the victorious Christian life that was purchased for you through Christ's death on the cross. You will pray with confidence using God's Word and God's promises as your foundation. You can claim those promises with confidence.

In this week's study you'll learn guidelines for effective prayer. If you haven't been studying the reflections on days six and seven, this would be a good week to start. It will reinforce your prayer life and prepare you to fight and win the battle through prayer.

## DAY 1: *The Right Reason Behind Prayer*

You pray for many reasons—some good, some inadequate. In difficult situations, you might pray hoping God will provide an escape hatch. In challenging circumstances, you might pray seeking God's guidance and grace. In times of need, you might pray for God's power, strength and wisdom. These and others are valid reasons for praying. They are not, however, the most important reason you should pray. John 14:13 tells us the most important reason for you to pray.

➤ Why should you pray?

Jesus promised to respond positively to your prayer when it meets the key criteria and gives God the glory.

➤ According to Matthew 6:33, what must you do for God to answer prayer?

Anything that promotes God's kingdom and righteousness insures God will receive glory. You can pray asking God to help you keep your First Place commitments with the focus on glorifying God.

➤ How can you obey 1 Corinthians 6:20?

God created you so that you can bring glory to Him through your life. Your physical body is one tool you can use to glorify God. Through everything you do, try to live in such a way that people think more highly of God because of what they see in you. If you want to bring your life under Christ's control in order to have a positive witness for Christ, you can ask God, with confidence, to help you keep your commitments. God knows if you intend to use your victory to bring Him glory! He also knows if you only want victory to satisfy selfish motives. Glorifying God with your life then strengthens the weapon of your personal testimony discussed last week. Not all prayer is effective and glorifies God.

➤ What are the two qualifications for effective prayer according to John 15:7?

1.

2.

Jesus encourages you to ask whatever you wish in prayer, confident you will receive what you ask, but you must remain close to God and allow His Word to dwell in you. The best way to keep God's Word continually in your heart is to memorize Scripture and use it in your daily life. Now read John 15:10 to see how you will know you are meeting the criteria for answered prayer.

> What is the criteria given by Jesus in John 15:10 for meeting answered prayer?

Obedience! Does that seem too difficult? Jesus modeled the obedient life for us on Earth. Through His obedience, He maintained an abiding relationship with His heavenly Father. Review Week One's memory verse, Deuteronomy 30:11. That is a promise you can count on.

> Write a prayer expressing your desire for God to help you be obedient and keep your First Place commitments this week for His glory, not your own.

Thank You, Lord, for the promise of answered prayer. Help me to be obedient to Your command so that I can bring glory to Your name.

Heavenly Father, help me to keep my focus on You and Your Word so that I may abide in You and know You abide in me.

# DAY 2: *Prayer in Difficult Times*

When you work with God's help to change areas of your life, you will face struggles. Victory is not instantaneous. Along the way you can get discouraged. Prayer becomes critically important for you in those difficult times.

➳ Read Psalm 107:19,20. What did the people described in this passage do in their time of trouble?

➳ What four things did God do in response to their action?

1.

2.

3.

4.

How wonderful to know that God will save you from distress! He has the power to heal and rescue you. The process begins when you cry out to God, seeking His help in times of trouble and difficulty. No matter what difficulty you face, you can bring that concern to God in prayer.

Even though you can't always be a pillar of strength when you need to be, God is there to uphold you and give you peace. He will give you the strength and courage necessary for any time of need. These times of difficulty and vulnerability are the times when Satan looks for a toehold. He looks for a tiny chink in the armor or a loose pebble in the dike. He's always on the prowl. Psalm 17:7,8 is a prayer of David that shows what to do when you pray.

➳ What did David ask of the Lord?

In times of difficulty and stress, you must seek God's face, listen to His Word and obey His commands.

➳ What does David say about God in Psalm 56:3,4?

⇒ How can you apply this to your own life?

Reread Jeremiah 33:3, this week's memory verse.

⇒ What must you do?

⇒ What will God show you?

Change produces pressure. It's easy to lose perspective and view your situation as an insurmountable problem. God understands. He wants you, in those times of stress, to call out to Him in prayer. You can tell Him your frustrations and fears. He, in turn, will affirm His plans to you. He'll remind you of His resources and power.

God responds when you call on Him through prayer. He will show you great and mighty things today as He works in your life. Focus your time of prayer today on any pressures and challenges you are facing as you confront the issues in your life as part of the First Place program.

Lord, You are my light and salvation; help me to be fearless as I battle the wiles of Satan.

Thank You, Lord Jesus, for giving me Your promises to hear me and give me an answer when I call on Your name.

# DAY 3: *The Powerful Name of Jesus*

Jesus offers His children blessings untold when they use His name.

≫ What is the promise found in John 14:13,14 when you pray in Jesus' name?




Praying in Jesus' name is far more than automatically tacking that phrase onto the end of your prayer. The right to pray in Jesus' name is a precious privilege that was purchased for us by Christ's death on the cross.

≫ The following verses provide insights into the power you can have when you pray in the name of Jesus. Read each verse and then fill in the missing words.

1. John 14:13—Jesus will do whatever_____

   _____.


2. John 14:14—You may_____

   _____and Jesus will do it.


3. John 15:16—Then the Father will _____

   _____.


4. John 16:23—The Father _____

   _____ask in Jesus' name.


5. John 16:24—Until now, you have not _____

   _____.

First John 3:22,23 provide additional insights on how you can receive answer to prayer. What are the two key commands in this passage?

1.


2.


When your life is characterized by obedience, believing in Jesus' name and loving one another, you receive wonderful blessings. When you live with the goal of pleasing God in all you do, He will delight in answering your prayers.

Because of Christ's death, you can pray as a child of God. When you pray in Jesus' name, you assume responsibility for praying in a manner consistent with His character. Ultimately, you seek to please and glorify Him. Praying in the name of Jesus is your privilege and your responsibility.

Father God, I know I am Your child. Help me to seek to please and glorify You in all that I do.

Lord, let my life be characterized by obedience in loving You and loving others.


# DAY 4: *Prayer and the Foundation of Faith*

God's Word must be in you as you are in Him. Build your life on this foundation and your life will be centered on God's truth and wisdom.

According to Deuteronomy 6:6,7, where does God want you to have His Word?




What does this mean to you and how would you know if you had done what He asked?

~ These verses picture people whose lives revolved around God's Word. What practical steps can you take to center your life on God's Word?

God wants you to believe He loves you and willingly provides all that you need. Satan tries to trip you at this point by injecting doubt in your mind. Satan scores a victory in your heart if he can cause you to question God's personal concern for you. Jesus wants you to stand securely in your relationship with God and pray with confidence. Your heavenly Father hears your prayers and will answer.

~ Hebrews 11:6 describes some basic principles for relating to God. When you pray, what two things are you affirming that you believe about God?

1.

2.

Your faith reveals what you believe about the object of your faith. When you pray in faith, you affirm the fact that you believe God exists and responds to those who seek Him. You affirm there is a spiritual realm of life that impacts your physical life. Through faith expressed in prayer, you express your desire to interact personally with God.

~ James 1:6,7 affirms the importance of faith in prayer.

1. When you pray, you must _____

_____.

2. The person who doubts is like _____

_____.

What should the one who prays doubtfully expect from the Lord?

Mark 9:14-27 relates a story of a man who sought Jesus' help.

What did Jesus tell the man who sought healing for his son (v. 23)?

What was the man's reply (v. 24)?

What was the result of the man's belief?

When you pray, believe and don't doubt. Affirm your belief in God and ask Him to help you with the areas in which you still struggle to believe. Be assured that you do have a God through whom all things are possible.

Lord God, help me to rely on You and to put my trust completely in You.

Father, help me to build my foundation of faith on You and Your Word.

# DAY 5: *Prayer and God's Will*

God is all-knowing and all-loving. He sees the past, the present *and* the future. He knows all that will happen and what everyone will do. God answers prayers according to His will. In 1 John 5:14,15 the apostle John explained the connections between God's will and answered prayer.

➤ How would you describe this connection between God's will and answered prayer?




You can pray confidently once you know God's will. Until you know God's will, your prayers can be presumptuous. God promises to answer your prayers when you align yourself with His will.

➤ Read Romans 12:1,2. How is God's will described in verse 2?




➤ If you struggle to know God's will in a particular situation, the following verses can help you discern His will:

Romans 8:26—What will the Holy Spirit do when you don't know how to pray?




2 Timothy 2:15—What skill must you develop in using the God's Word?




James 4:3—What wrong motives must you avoid in prayer?




Trust God to reveal His will to you through the Bible. Satan will not wait for you to run for your Bible before he hits you with temptation. God encourages you repeatedly in Scripture to memorize and meditate on His Word. This is the prime reason for memorizing Scripture each week with your First Place Bible studies. Exercise with your CD or cassette, listen to it in the car or as you work. Write His words on your heart.

➤ According to Psalm 37:31, what benefit will you experience when you have God's Word in your heart?

➤ Read Psalm 119:105. What place does the Word of God have in your life?

➤ In James 1:22-25, what is the person who listens to the Word but doesn't do it compared to?

➤ What is the gift of remembering and obeying God's Word?

➤ What does it mean for you personally to read, learn and obey the Word of God?

 Lord God, help me to pray with pure motives and without any doubts.

Oh, Father God, I pray for Your Holy Spirit to help me find and understand Your will for my life.

# DAY 6: *Reflections*

In this week's study you have learned several guidelines for prayer. Not only must you believe that God promises to answer prayer, but you must also have His Word in you and obey His commands. Last week you learned how prayer keeps you in constant communion with God and gives divine power to your life. Through prayer you can reach the ultimate goal of true intimacy with God.

Praying Scripture gives your prayers extra ammunition in your warfare with Satan. Spend time talking with God in a conversational way as you study His Word, and your relationship will grow. His will is revealed as you become closer to Him and read His Word.

God's will for your life is for you to love Him, obey Him and serve Him, and then He will give you great and wonderful things and untold blessings. This does not mean that you will never be tempted, never have trials or never know sorrow. It does mean that when temptations, trials and sorrows do come, you will be prepared to go through them with God's mercy, love and strength.

When you pray asking God to give you the power you need to obey Him today, He will answer and give you what you need for today. Then you will live in a way that pleases Him.

In your prayer time this week, seek to follow His will and obey Him. In so doing you will overcome the strongholds in your life.

Father God, You have promised that I will overcome my strongholds because the One who is in me is greater than the one who is the world. Help me to trust in You and Your Word (see 1 John 4:4).

Father God, protect me by the power of Your name (see John 17:11).

My Father, please help me to be on my guard, stand firm in the faith, be a person of courage, be strong and do everything in love (see 1 Corinthians 16:13).

# DAY 7: *Reflections*

You have learned guidelines for effective prayer. One of those guidelines involved having the proper reasons or motivation. One of those reasons is to bring glory to the Father. God promised to give you what you need if you seek Him first. Praying Scripture brings glory to God as you read His Word and make it a part of your life.

Your physical body as well as your mind can bring glory to Him demonstrated in the life you live through Him. You seek His will for your life as you read and study His Word and then make it a part of your life. Memorizing Scripture gives you guidance as you make decisions and live your life each day. Your actions reflect your relationship with the Lord. How can He bless you beyond measure if you do not know Him?

His Word teaches you to love others as yourself and to love the Lord your God with every part of your being. You show that love by your obedience to His will and keeping His Word in your heart. Search the Word, hide it in your heart and then pray His Word. Last week you read how Beth Moore believes that prayer is one of your two most powerful weapons against Satan—the other is God's Word.

God knows the difficulty you face as you live in the world. He knows how easily you slip and fall. His Word makes you secure and stable and gives you a solid foundation on which to stand. Having stability in a shaky world is a tremendous benefit! Your best defense against temptation is to memorize His Word and meditate on it.

Focus on the following verses in prayer as you seek security in God's Word and build a solid foundation for your faith:

Father, help me to understand that Satan, the ultimate thief, comes only to steal and kill and destroy; You came so that I could have life and have it more abundantly (see John 10:10).

Jesus, may my prayers always be in Your name so that You will answer and bring glory to the Father. You promise to do whatever I ask in Your name (see John 14:13,14).

Father God, do not let me be like a wave tossed about by the wind because I doubt. Help me to believe without doubt so that I may receive Your blessings (see James 1:6,7).

Lord, I call on Your name so that You will answer and show me great and unsearchable things that I do not know (see Jeremiah 33:3).

# GROUP PRAYER REQUESTS  TODAY'S DATE:_____

| NAME | REQUEST | RESULTS |
|------|---------|---------|
|      |         |         |
|      |         |         |
|      |         |         |
|      |         |         |
|      |         |         |
|      |         |         |
|      |         |         |
|      |         |         |
|      |         |         |
|      |         |         |
|      |         |         |
|      |         |         |
|      |         |         |
|      |         |         |

# MOTIVES AND ATTITUDES

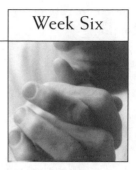

### MEMORY VERSE
*We make it our goal to please him, whether*
*we are at home in the body or away from it.*
2 Corinthians 5:9

Two internal factors will influence your success in the First Place program: your motives and your attitudes. Here are two working definitions you can use:

- Motives—the inner drives that compel you to act in a certain way. Motives explain why you do something.
- Attitudes—opinions or beliefs you hold about the things you do. Attitudes explain how you feel about what you do.

In this week's study, you'll learn about the motives that God can bless and use. You'll learn about attitudes that will make it easier for you to reach your goals in the First Place program.

## DAY 1: *The Motive Behind the Action*

Thomas à Kempis said, "Man sees your actions, but God your motives." People may focus on your actions and appearance, but God looks deeper.

➤ According to 1 Samuel 16:7, on what does God focus?

God focuses on what is inside your heart or what is behind the things you do. To God it's not enough that you do good things, the right things. God cares about your motives. He considers what prompts you to take action.

You do things for many reasons. Sometimes those reasons are not pleasing to God. Scripture shows some of the negative motives that do not please God.

➤ Read the following Scripture verses and match them to the negative motive:

a. Proverbs 16:5        _____ selfish ambition

b. Proverbs 16:18       _____ vain conceit

c. 1 Corinthians 13:4   _____ haughty spirit

d. Philippians 2:3      _____ envy

                        _____ proud in heart

                        _____ boastfulness

➤ When you made the decision to join First Place, what motives influenced you? Be as specific and honest as you can and tell why you set a particular goal such as losing weight or feeling better.

Often pride is behind the motivation to join a program such as First Place. Pride in yourself and how you look to others is often the first motive. You think of how you will look and feel and what you will do once you lose weight. Personal pride may even motivate you to change your lifestyle and add healthy food, exercise and even Bible study; but is it pride in what you can accomplish or is it what God can do for you? God has strong feelings about pride.

➤ According to James 4:6, what does God do to prideful people?

➤ What does God do for humble people?


➤ In what category are you right now?

The First Place program is about more than weight loss. The nine commitments lead to a well-rounded life in Christ. Memorizing Scripture, Bible study and prayer bring you closer to spiritual well-being in an intimate relationship with God. Exercise and the Live-It program give you physical well-being. The encouragement of others and your weekly meetings bring emotional support. All together these commitments give you a better mental attitude. The First Place program produces balanced living.

God resists the proud and the humble receive grace. Confess any pride to God and trust Him to give you grace. Express your need for Him and trust Him to provide the motivation you need to reach the goals you set for this session.

Thank You, Lord, for loving me. Give me the right attitude and motives as I seek to improve my health. May it all be for Your glory.

Dear God, tear down my pride and bring me closer to You and let Your grace abound in me.


# DAY 2: *Positive Motivation*

With two minutes left in the football game and his team leading by three points, the coach warned his quarterback, "Don't pass the ball under any circumstances." However, once in the game the quarterback forgot the warning and threw a pass. The ball sailed directly into the hands of the opposing team's safety who caught it on the run. The safety ran toward the goal line and apparent victory. At the last second, he was tackled on the five-yard line by the quarterback who had thrown the pass. The clock ran out. The game was saved. Later, the two coaches spoke.

"How in the world did your quarterback catch my safety?" the losing coach asked.

"That's easy," the other coach replied, "Your safety was running for a touchdown. My quarterback was running for his life!"

You must be motivated if you hope to accomplish difficult tasks. The question you need to answer is, What motivation is appropriate for a Christian?

As you read the following verses, answer the questions and rate the degree to which your life demonstrates that positive motive by circling a number:

>> 2 Corinthians 5:9—What should be your goal?

This motive is weak in my life.　　This motive is strong in my life.

| 1 | 2 | 3 | 4 | 5 |

>> Romans 12:1—How should you present your body to God?

This motive is weak in my life.　　This motive is strong in my life.

| 1 | 2 | 3 | 4 | 5 |

>> Philippians 1:20—What should occur in your life, no matter what you do?

This motive is weak in my life.　　This motive is strong in my life.

| 1 | 2 | 3 | 4 | 5 |

➣ According to Philippians 2:3, what should you avoid in your motivation for service?

➣ What should your motivation be?

➣ What did Paul mean in Philippians 1:21?

Throughout the New Testament God encourages and motivates us to continue to give Him glory. Your motives for action then should be to please God, to express worship to Him and to exalt Christ through your body. God will support those whose actions are prompted by those motives! He will help you live your life with motives that please Him.

 Lord, be merciful to me and motivate me to live my life to glorify and worship You.

Thank You, Lord Jesus, for giving clear instruction in how to live. Motivate me to present my body as a living sacrifice for You.

# DAY 3: *Sustaining Motivation*

When your life is driven by selfish pride, God resists you. When your life is driven by positive, spiritual motives, God empowers you. To be effective, motivation must last.

➤ Philippians 2:13 explains that God will work in your life to help you in practical ways. What does God do for you?

➤ This verse shows how God give us the power to do things that please Him. God will give you the *want to* and the *can do*. While you have been involved in the First Place program, in what ways has God increased your *want to*?

➤ What is your motivation to make changes in your life?

➤ In what ways have you noticed your *can do* increasing since you began the First Place program?

God provides the power you need to accomplish His will in your life. He will work in your life and give you the desire and the power to live a healthy life. He will give you all you need to make the necessary changes in your life.

➤ What does Philippians 4:19 mean to you in the light of God's provision in your life with First Place?

➤ How can Philippians 3:13,14 motivate you to continue toward your goals in First Place?

Thank God for giving you the *want to*. He will increase your desire to eat and live right, and He will help you to solve the problems that come your way. He will increase your *can do*. Trust Him to give you the power you need to make the difficult changes in your life.

 Father God, You know the desires of my heart and the changes I need to make. Give me the strength, O Father, to make the changes and follow Your will for my life.

Lord, be with me each day as I face temptation. Motivate me to be obedient to Your commands.

# DAY 4: *Christ and Your Attitude*

Your attitude toward life influences the results you achieve in life. A. W. Tozer said, "Things are for us only what we hold them to be. Which is to say that our attitude toward things is likely in the long run to be more important than the things themselves."

➽ How would you describe your attitude about the First Place program and the changes you are making in your life?

You should strive to maintain a cheerful attitude that gives glory to God. You must resist any desire to moan about the things you can no longer do. Your conscious decision to be positive and cheerful protects your Christian witness. An unhappy, disgruntled Christian is a poor testimony to the goodness of God. Happiness is a choice you make.

➽ Colossians 3:23 explains the attitude that should characterize everything you do in life. Rewrite this verse in your own words.

By monitoring your thought life, you insure that the attitudes you develop will be positive. In Philippians 4:8 Paul listed positive thoughts that you should nurture.

≫ Use the following chart to focus on each positive thought mentioned in this passage. In the space to the right, beside each positive thought, write an opposite, negative thought to be avoided. Two are shown as examples.

| Positive Thoughts (Philippians 4:8) | Negative Thoughts (The Opposite of Philippians 4:8) |
|---|---|
| True | *Something base, low* |
| Noble | |
| Right | |
| Pure | |
| Lovely | |
| Admirable | |
| Excellent | *Inferior, cheap, shoddy* |
| Praiseworthy | |

Everything you do in life should reflect your desire to please Christ. You live for Christ, and you are successful if Christ is pleased. Your positive thoughts please God.

≫ What changes would occur in your thoughts and attitudes toward your problems if you could honestly say, "I'm doing this for Jesus Christ that He may be glorified through my life."

God will help you deal with your problems and change your habits. He can turn your life into a testimony of His power and grace.

Lord God, I ask that You fill my mind with positive thoughts that will help me fulfill Your will for my life.

Father, when negative thoughts and attitudes threaten to come in and defeat me, give me Your words to fill my mind and resist the temptations that will come.

## DAY 5: *An Attitude Shaped by Thanksgiving*

Clement Stone observed, "There is little difference in people, but that little difference makes a big difference. The little difference is attitude. The big difference is whether it is positive or negative." You can choose positive attitudes that strengthen your life. Christians have so many positive things on which to focus. Christians, more than other people, have no excuse for negativism.

➢ You can nurture thankfulness in your life. The following verses reveal insights about an attitude of thanksgiving:

1 Thessalonians 5:18—How can you apply this principle of thanksgiving to your work in the First Place program?

Psalm 28:7—What positive truths in this verse can you apply to your life as you work to change your habits?

Romans 8:28—How does this verse apply to your present experience in First Place?

1 Corinthians 15:57,58—How can these verses motivate you to have a positive attitude?

1 Timothy 4:4,5—Why are you to accept the things in your life with thanksgiving?

God promises to use the pressure of difficult times in your life to bring positive results. In light of all that God does for you, your minimum response must be thanksgiving. Always be thankful for all God has done and will do for you. Being negative and discouraged becomes difficult when you focus on all He has done for you. Focus, therefore, on the things God has done and thank Him for His blessings.

 Oh, Father God, forgive my negative attitudes and give me positive thoughts as I focus on Your many blessings in my life.

Heavenly Father, I seek to be positive as I focus on You and give thanks for the many blessings You bestow on my life.

## DAY 6: *Reflections*

In this week's study you have learned about the importance of having a positive attitude in all that you do, especially in your thoughts concerning changing your habits. You control your attitude by what you think. By monitoring your thought life, you can insure that the attitudes you develop will be positive.

Memorizing Scripture gives you the foundation for your godly thoughts. When you face temptations, negative thoughts and poor attitudes, focus on God's love. Quoting a passage of Scripture is a wonderful way to automatically replace a negative thought with a positive one. Positive thoughts help you think about the truths that will build your life, encourage you and help you reach your spiritual goals. When your life and thoughts are filled with the positive, the negative doesn't have room to come in.

Here then is another excellent reason for hiding God's Word in your heart and mind. Prayer using Scripture as its focus helps you keep your eyes on Jesus. With your eyes on Him, you can't help but think positively.

Father God, You have promised to give me a new heart and put a new spirit within me. You will take out my heart of stone and give me one of flesh to love and serve You. Fill me with Your thoughts (see Ezekiel 36:26).

Father God, I know that my fears of failure are not from You because You have not given me a spirit of fear, but a spirit of power and love and a sound mind. Help me to reject those fears (see 2 Timothy 1:7).

My Father, show me Your ways, teach me your paths, guide me in Your truth and teach me—for You are my God, my Savior, and my hope is in You all day long (see Psalm 25:4,5).

## DAY 7: Reflections

God has promised to give you what you need if you seek Him first. Remember that praying Scripture brings glory to God as you read His Word and make it a part of your life.

God wants your life to attract attention. Christ works in you, transforming your life until you become increasingly like Him. When others see you, they see a reflection of Christ. If people know you are a Christian, yet observe you doing or saying things Christ would not do or say, they wonder what difference being a Christian makes. They may watch even more closely when they know you are going through a challenging time. They want to know if Christ really does make a difference in your life.

When you are going through a particularly trying time, responding positively may be difficult. You may even rationalize and blame your attitudes and actions on the difficulties you're having, but God never gives you permission to be negative. Instead, He provides the power for you to respond cheerfully to others by using His Word. Don't let negative thoughts and actions become a stronghold for you. Many verses tell you about responding to others and having a positive attitude. Search out verses and commit them to memory; then use them when you are facing a difficult situation.

》 Proverbs 15:13,15,30 will get you started on your assignment to find verses to help when you need to be positive in your thoughts and attitudes. Write a short prayer using these verses, asking God to give you a positive attitude.

God will continue to work in your life daily when you call on Him in prayer. The following Scripture verses will help you develop positive attitudes this week:

Father, help me to respond with pleasant words to others because they are a honeycomb, sweet to the soul and healing to the bones (see Proverbs 16:24).

Father, help me to guard my mouth and tongue and keep myself from calamity. Help me to speak only in a positive way for You (see Proverbs 21:23).

Father God, let the Holy Spirit teach what I should say when I am feeling discouraged and others seem to plot against me (see Luke 12:12).

Lord, help me make it my goal to please You, whether I am at home in the body or away from it (see 2 Corinthians 5:9).

# GROUP PRAYER REQUESTS   TODAY'S DATE:_____

| NAME | REQUEST | RESULTS |
|------|---------|---------|
|      |         |         |
|      |         |         |
|      |         |         |
|      |         |         |
|      |         |         |
|      |         |         |
|      |         |         |
|      |         |         |
|      |         |         |
|      |         |         |
|      |         |         |
|      |         |         |
|      |         |         |
|      |         |         |

# RUN TO WIN

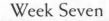
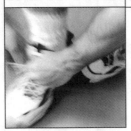

## MEMORY VERSE

*However, I consider my life worth nothing to me
if only I may finish the race and complete the task the
Lord Jesus has given me—the task of
testifying to the gospel of God's grace.*

Acts 20:24

The Christian life is a race. When you became a Christian, you entered
the race. Are you still in the race? How well are you running?

Perhaps you've realized the strongholds and temptations in your life
have hindered your ability to run the race. Congratulations. You've taken
an important step. Becoming a part of the First Place program was a turning point.

In this week's study, you'll learn more about the Christian race. You'll
learn principles that will help you run well, finish the race and win the
prize.

## DAY 1: *A Race to Run*

Hebrews 12:1 pictures the Christian life in vivid images. The race of faith
is cast as a grueling marathon. As you run, a great cloud of witnesses is
looking on. They watch with anticipation to see if you will complete the
course and finish the faith.

➤ In the context of this verse, who are these witnesses that watch you
run the race?

All the saints who have gone on before you now watch to see how
you run the race. They are there to encourage and motivate you.

➤ Think about the way you have lived your Christian life. If you had to compare your life with an actual running event, how would it be classified? Check the race category that might characterize your life.

☐ Spectator—watch while others run

☐ Walkathon—walk while others run

☐ Fun Run—run until it begins to hurt; then stop

☐ Sprint—start fast, but burn out quickly

☐ Marathon—keep a steady pace; go the distance

➤ Why did you make that choice?

God has called you to run a marathon for Christ. If you attempt to view the Christian life in any other way, you dilute the vital faith Christ wants you to enjoy.

Hebrews 11 is the Hall of Faith for the saints of the Old Testament. Read Hebrews 12:1 again. Those about whom Paul writes in chapter 11 are part of the cloud of witnesses mentioned in this verse.

➤ How does having these faithful saints watch your race of faith make you feel?

In 1 Corinthians 9:25, you'll find another important athletic principle that illustrates the faith race.

➤ What image did Paul use in 1 Corinthians 9:25 to illustrate this principle?

Before athletes were allowed to participate in the games, they had to train for their event. Athletes who did not train could not keep up the pace. Before becoming a part of First Place, did you consider strict training essential to your Christian life?

➤ From the following list, choose the answer that best describes your *past* attitude:

- [ ] Becoming a Christian is all that is necessary.
- [ ] I attend church and assume that is enough spiritual training.
- [ ] Spiritual training is for super-Christians, ministers and missionaries.
- [ ] I want to develop my spiritual life, but I don't know how to start.
- [ ] I'm committed to developing my spiritual life and I work at it every day.

➤ Explain your answer.

As a Christian you have an incredible heritage of faith. As you run the race God has set for you, be encouraged by the living testimony of the men and women who have gone before you. When you consider the price they paid to live for Christ, you will be motivated to deal with any difficult area of your life that is hindering your ability to live for Jesus Christ.

➤ What are the strongholds or problems in your life that have hindered your ability to run the spiritual race God has set before you?

➤ What price are you willing to pay for the strict training you need to run your race?

Many Christians believe their spiritual race can be run with minimal training. As a result, they live for Christ the best they can, never truly understanding why they are often frustrated. God designed the Christian life as a life of victory, but it is a life that demands you to train spiritually and develop your life for Christ.

Dear God, give me the desire and motivation to run my spiritual race in ways that will be pleasing to You.

Father, I want to develop my spiritual life and grow closer to You. Help me grow in ability as I run the race of faith.

# DAY 2: *A Prize to Win*

A little boy got a new archery set. His grandfather stacked some bales of hay behind the barn and helped the boy learn to use his bow and arrows. After some practice, the boy could shoot the arrows in the general direction of the hay bales. His grandfather then proceeded to fasten a multicolored target to the hay bales. The boy watched him and said, "Grandpa, I don't want to use that target. I like it when I shoot and you say 'good,' no matter where my arrows land." It is the same in your spiritual life—God has given you a target to aim for: the life of Christ.

➤ How do you feel about the spiritual training you've been getting in the First Place program?

The work you do in the First Place program is spiritual training. Initially you should focus on bringing only one area of your life under Christ's control. Once you experience victory in that area, you should move on to other areas that need Christ's control.

➤ According to 1 Corinthians 9:24, with what attitude should you live your spiritual life?

God wants you to be spiritually competitive. You aren't racing against others, but God has called you to a personal race of faith. You are accountable only for how you run *your* race.

➤ What does Philippians 3:14 say about your future spiritual prize?




God allows you to live on Earth knowing that one day you will complete your earthly race and stand before Him in heaven to receive your prize. On that day, God will evaluate the way you have run. Your goal should be to hear Him say, "Well done, faithful runner. I am pleased."

Galatians 2:20 informs us of a dimension of the spiritual prize you can enjoy now.

➤ What is your reward in this present life?




➤ What is Christ doing in your life right now? In what ways have you experienced Him living in you?




For the Christian, Christ is the prize. He works in your life, giving you the desire and the power to live in a way that pleases Him. He empowers you in practical ways such as helping you to reach your goals and living a healthier life. Incredible as it seems, the God of the universe does work in your life. This is the prize you can enjoy now!

In Acts 20:24, your memory verse, Paul explained the task he hoped to complete in his own life.

➤ What is the task given to you according to this verse?

➤ In what ways is God using your training in First Place to help you share with others the gospel of God's grace?

With strict training you will reach the finish line and claim the prize that God has for all who follow Him and are obedient to His commands.

Lord, thank You for the work You are doing in me and for giving me such a great prize. Help me to continue to live for You and run my race faithfully to the end.

Thank You, Lord Jesus, for loving me and dying for me so that I may live with You when my race is finished.

## DAY 3: A Danger of Disqualification

Playing games with children can be frustrating. Rules often are invented (or changed) as the game progresses. "That's not how I play," someone might say; and an appeal to the official rules generally does no good. It doesn't work that way in the spiritual life; we cannot decide to make up our own spiritual rules for our lives.

➤ What does 2 Timothy 2:5 say about the rules for a race?

➤ According to 2 Timothy 3:16,17, how can you know the rules for the spiritual race?

➤ What are the four purposes of Scripture?

1.

2.

3.

4.

All Scripture is inspired by God and useful to us. Look at how much He provides for you to keep you on the right track and in the right lane in your spiritual race.

➤ According to 1 Corinthians 9:27, why can't you simply live your Christian life any way you choose?

➤ Does the possibility of disqualification concern you?

➤ What was John's purpose, according to 1 John 5:13, for writing his first epistle?

➤ What does this verse mean to you?

In 1 Corinthians 3:10-15, Paul describes his work for Christ as if he were building a house.

➤ How will that building be tested?

You cannot earn salvation through what you do, but you have the opportunity to express love to Christ by what you do! God will help you live all areas in your life in such a way that your life will be a gift of love you can offer Him.

 Father God, help me to build my life on a solid foundation based on Your love for me through Your death on the cross.

Lord, help me to use Your Word to teach, train, correct and rebuke myself so that I will run the race based on Your rules and win the prize You have for me.

## DAY 4: *Staying on Course*

God has a race marked out for you. God wants to fill your life with positive experiences, but sometimes the negatives creep in. He wants you to run with perseverance, joy and determination to succeed.

➤ According to 1 Corinthians 9:26, what are the two negative examples of running a race?

1.

2.

In your spiritual life, you need to be like the runners who run with a clear sense of direction. Be like a fighter who boxes for real—not just shadow boxing. Obviously, God intends for you to accomplish a clear purpose in your spiritual life. Sometimes you might struggle to know the direction God has planned for you, but you can know the overall course of your race.

Anytime God works in your life, you have an opportunity to testify to others about Him. People long to know that God exists and that He works in their lives. Your responsibility is to tell them by sharing your own experience. In 2 Timothy 4:7,8, Paul reflected on the way he had lived for Jesus Christ.

➤ What changes do you need to make so that you can stand at the end of your life and say "I finished the race"?

➤ When the race is finished, the course complete, what will be your reward?

➤ According to Romans 8:29, what does God want to accomplish in your life?

➤ How does 2 Corinthians 5:17 describe the changes God is making in you?

God began transforming you into the image of Christ when you became a Christian. He will not stop working on you until you are transformed into the image of Jesus Christ. Such radical transformation involves every area of your life. In the First Place program you will focus on all four aspects of your life: physical, spiritual, emotional and mental. God will transform these areas of your life when you seek His help and guidance. You are a work in progress—always under construction. You have the right to the victory in overcoming the world. You are a conqueror.

According to 1 John 5:4,5, who is it that overcomes the world?

God is doing a wonderful work in your life and is helping you become a new creation—inside and outside!

Lord God, thank You for transforming my life and making me a new creation.

Father, continue Your work in me and motivate me so that I will stay on the course and finish the race You set for me.

## DAY 5: *Perseverance Until the End*

Hebrews 12:1,2 provides important insights for running a long-distance race for Christ.

What two steps are required for success in this race?

1.

2

As a Christian you should use both steps to focus on many areas of your life. In the First Place program, you learn how to eat in healthier ways, memorize Scripture, encourage others in their struggles, pray and study God's Word in your efforts to become closer to Him. Use these steps to develop spiritual maturity in all areas of your life.

What is one particular area of your life that may be hindering you, something that is not sin yet still needs to be set aside so you can run your spiritual race (for example, rationalizing eating habits, making excuses for not exercising or being too busy for quiet time and Bible study)? What can you do to get rid of this hindrance?

➤ Is there some element of your spiritual life that could be classified as sin that entangles you (for example, pride, sarcasm, resentment, anger, impatience with others)? Name it and explain one action you can take to get rid of this sin.

➤ What does Romans 6:12,13 tell you about these weaknesses or sins?

➤ What encouragement do 1 Corinthians 10:13 and Hebrews 2:17,18; 4:14-16 offer about your ability to persevere and win the race set before you?

➤ What is the promise found in Romans 8:37,38?

➤ What does Romans 15:4 mean to you as you run your race?

With God's help, you will finish the race and attain the prize of eternal life.

Oh, Father God, take all the sins that threaten to entangle me and let me live my life for You in a way that is pleasing and acceptable in Your eyes.

Thank You, heavenly Father, for making me a conqueror and giving me the victory that overcomes the world.

# DAY 6: *Reflections*

In this week's study you have learned about the importance of running the race God marked out for you and giving testimony of your faith in the gospel and of the grace of the Lord Jesus Christ. As you focus on this week's memory verse, ask God how to put that memory verse to work in your life. Think of ways you can give testimony to the gospel of God's grace. Memorizing and sharing verses with others gives you the opportunity to share important biblical truths with those around you.

While God is doing His work in your life, let others see and know how your life is changing and what God is doing for you. By adhering to the strict training required for a successful race, you will have the victory and others will see your success.

No matter what the stronghold is in your life, no matter how big or how small it is, God shows in His Word how to overcome it. With the Word of God and prayer as your primary weapons, you will overcome every stronghold and be victorious in your race. In Beth Moore's book *Praying God's Word*, she describes how the two mightiest weapons—God's Word and prayer—are like "two sticks of dynamite" that are a powerful force against any stronghold you may have.[1]

In the chapter titled "Overcoming Addiction," Moore says that God can set you free of your addictions—whether they be substances or behaviors. However, God requires from you time, trust and cooperation. Release won't come in a day or even several weeks, but it will come if you persevere, stay on course and focus your eyes on Jesus Christ. The harder the lesson, the more long-lasting it will be.[2]

Prayer using Scripture as your focus will help to keep you on course. The following prayers are adapted from Moore's book:

 Search me, O God, and know my heart; test me and know my anxious thoughts. See if there is any offensive way in me, and lead me in the way everlasting (see Psalm 139:23,24).

O Lord, cause my soul to yearn for You in the night and long for You in the morning (see Isaiah 26:9).

Father, who can separate me from the love of Christ? Can trouble or hardship or persecution or famine or nakedness or danger or sword? No, in all these things I am more than a conqueror through You because You love me (see Romans 8:35,37).[3]

# DAY 7: *Reflections*

Since the focus this week is on running the race and following the course God has set for you, think of ways you can serve Him and testify of His grace in your life. Keeping a prayer journal not only gives you a place to list the prayer needs of the day or week, but it also gives you a place to list the answers to prayer as they come. Your prayer journal is also a good place to write down Scripture verses that are a blessing to you. This will help you memorize verses that you can directly apply to your daily walk with Him.

When your relationship with Jesus Christ is on a level that brings you closer to Him each day, He provides the needed stamina, strength and desire to endure to the end. His Word is full of promises and hope for a future that will only bring good in your life. He will also provide the weapons for you to fight your spiritual battles, and He always provides a way of escape when you are tempted by Satan or the desires of the world.

In addition to the assigned memory verse for the week, look for another meaningful verse in your Bible study and commit it to memory. Write it in your prayer journal or start your own memory-verse cards. If you are reading Beth Moore's book, look up the verses she uses in her prayers and write a prayer of your own. Using God's Word in prayer will make it come alive for you and become your own.

By now you should be more comfortable with Scripture memory. If you still feel it's too difficult for you, let's review how you can make memorization a little easier.

1.  Write the verse down several times and read it aloud as you write it.

2.  Personalize the verse by putting your name in key places and by putting it into your own words. This will give you ownership of the verse and help you apply it.

3.  Seek to understand the verse. Always read the verse in its context. Study the verse to understand its meaning.

4.  In order to learn the reference, always repeat it before and after each time you say the verse. This will help to *glue* the reference to the first and last few words of the verse.

Learning and using God's Word in prayer gives you power to defeat Satan at every turn, just as Jesus defeated him in the wilderness. The power of God's Word will tear down any stronghold that is keeping you from a full, intimate relationship with your Lord Jesus Christ. The verse cards and CD/cassette are further aids as you seek to commit God's Word to memory.

God will continue to work in your life daily when You call on Him in prayer. Here are more prayers based on Scripture to help you this week.

Lord God, You are my stronghold in time of trouble. Help me. Deliver me from the wicked and save me because I take refuge in You (see Psalm 37:39,40).

Father, strengthen my faith for You have said that without faith it is impossible to please You; for he who comes to You, O God, must believe that You exist and that You will reward those who earnestly seek You (see Hebrews 11:6).

Father God, I cast my cares on You and You will sustain me; You will never permit the righteous to be moved. Keep me steadfast and true as I depend on You (see Psalm 55:22).

Lord, my life is worthless to me if I don't finish the race and complete the task You have given me of testifying to the gospel of Your wonderful grace (see Acts 20:24).

Notes
1. Beth Moore, *Praying God's Word* (Nashville, TN. Broadman and Holman, 2000), p. 6.
2. Ibid., pp 127, 128.
3. Ibid., pp. 131, 134, 137.

# GROUP PRAYER REQUESTS  TODAY'S DATE:_____

| NAME | REQUEST | RESULTS |
|------|---------|---------|
|      |         |         |
|      |         |         |
|      |         |         |
|      |         |         |
|      |         |         |
|      |         |         |
|      |         |         |
|      |         |         |
|      |         |         |
|      |         |         |
|      |         |         |
|      |         |         |
|      |         |         |

# OVERCOMING TEMPTATION

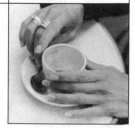

MEMORY VERSE
*"Not by might nor by power, but by my Spirit,"*
*says the LORD Almighty.*
Zechariah 4:6

God loves you and wants you to be successful. He will not, however, rearrange your surroundings, so you will not be tempted to give in to your strongholds.

In today's society, you will frequently find yourself in situations where you may be confronted by unwholesome things. Television shows, movies, music, food, parties and even church social gatherings may offer temptations you have struggled with in the past. Holidays, social events and family gatherings always include opportunities to overindulge. Eating, it seems, is the great American pastime!

God can give you victory in the midst of your circumstances whatever they may be. He wants to work in your life from the inside out. He wants to make you strong enough to resist temptation. In this week's study, you'll learn how to draw on the power of Christ to overcome temptation.

## DAY 1: *Depending on God*

In 1 Corinthians 10:13, we learn how temptation is a common occurrence and happens to everyone. Each of us has our own areas of strong temptation. Yours may be food; others may be tempted by alcohol, lying, using hurtful words, stubbornness, anger, a quick temper or pride. Whatever your temptation, God is with you and will help you overcome it.

➤ First Corinthians 10:13 contains two important principles. Complete the following sentences:

1. God will not let you _____.

2. When you are tempted, _____.

*God is faithful.* This means you can count on God to consistently do two things: monitor the level of temptation in your life and provide exits when temptations come.

➤ To what degree can you make the statement "God is faithful to me" about your Christian life in general? Give specific examples.

➤ How have you experienced God's faithfulness in helping you deal with temptation?

God sets the limits on the temptations that come into your life. This is what Paul explained in 1 Corinthians 10:13. God monitors the temptation levels, insuring the pressure on you never exceeds what you can resist.

➤ Check the boxes beside what you believe are principles suggested by "he will not let you be tempted beyond what you can bear."

☐ All temptation in my life is within acceptable limits. I *can* resist it.

☐ If I *can* resist any temptation in my life, I *should* resist it.

☐ If I *should* resist the temptation in my life, God expects me to do so.

☐ If I fail to resist temptation, I must assume responsibility for my actions.

All four of the statements contain valid principles. But God does not simply stand by and demand that you resist temptation on your own.

He is actively involved in helping you battle temptation. Notice that God provides the way out of temptation so that you can resist—and escape.

God doesn't expect you to yield to temptation and then rationalize and make excuses for your behavior. Remember the trouble that Eve had when she gave in to temptation and then led Adam into temptation. That temptation wasn't from God. He doesn't tempt you. Satan tempts you, but God puts on a restraint and won't allow you to be tempted over what you can bear. God did promise to provide an escape out of temptation. God did *not* promise the following:

- Easy-to-take escape routes
- Multiple opportunities to escape

Life would be much simpler if either or both of the above statements were true. God will respond faithfully to you as you face temptation in your life. Pray and ask Him to show you the way of escape.

Dear God, thank You for loving me enough to provide an escape route when temptations come into my life. Help me to be faithful and to listen to You

Father, I seek Your guidance in all areas of my life because You have promised to help me overcome any and every stronghold I have in my life.

## DAY 2: *Fully Known by God*

God gave us a wonderful promise when He said we won't be tempted beyond what we can bear. That promise affirms that God knows our limits and insures that temptation remains within the range we can resist.

➤ What does Psalm 139:1-4 tell you that God knows about you?

The Bible says God has searched and knows you. He knows your thoughts and everything about you, even how you think and feel. He is intimately involved with you. No area in your life is unfamiliar to Him.

➤ How do you feel about the fact that God knows you so fully? Mark an X on each of the three lines below indicating how you feel:

Good _____ Bad

Excited _____ Scared

Comfortable _____ Uncomfortable

➤ In each of the following verses, who does God say He knows and cares for?

Nahum 1:7

John 10:27

2 Timothy 2:19

How incredible that the God of the universe knows you. He knows your ways. He cares for you. He guides your life like a gentle shepherd. Nothing in your life surprises Him—including the struggles you have in overcoming temptation. In every area, God faithfully monitors the activities of you life to insure that you succeed. If you do have a problem with overeating or eating the wrong foods, turn that over to God, too. He cares about you in a way that no one else does.

➤ What is the promise found in John 15:5-7?

This means that any problem you have concerning the commitments you made to First Place can be turned over to God. Through the Holy Spirit, He will give you strength and comfort to do all you need to be successful. It won't be easy. Sometimes the end result won't be what you expected, but the decision to make a change will bring rewards.

Working on these Bible studies, meeting weekly with your First Place group and being close to God on a daily basis will change your life. Any weight loss that comes with it is serendipitous. Our prayer for you as you work on these studies and attend your group meetings is that you will find a closer, more intimate relationship with Him. When you do, resisting temptation will become easier for you.

Spend time talking to God about your strongholds and the things that tempt you most. When you confess your areas of weakness to Him, He is faithful to listen and to guide you. The more fully you know Him, the more you will see how much He cares about even the details of your life. Give the Lord *complete* control, and you will have a freedom like you've never experienced before.

 Lord, You know my very being, every weakness, every strength. Guide me and instruct me in Your ways. Thank You for Your faithfulness.

Heavenly Father, help me know You more fully through Your words in Scripture and through prayer.

# DAY 3: *Battling the Imagination*

When you are faced with a temptation, the first area the enemy attacks is your thoughts. Before you can do anything, you must first imagine yourself doing it. Jeremiah 7:24 shows what happens when you do not pay attention to God.

➤ What happens when you stubbornly follow the leading of your thoughts and imagination?

It is your privilege to base your life on God's Word and His leadership in your life. God's truth provides a solid foundation that keeps you from slipping backward in your life. Thoughts must be filtered through God's truth. Imagination must be put to the test. You may think about an action, even enjoy the thought, but you do not have to act on what you think.

Second Corinthians 10:4,5 provides a strategy for getting control over your thoughts and gaining power over temptation.

➤ What strategy is provided? Complete the following statements:

1. You have _____  _____ to demolish strongholds.

2. You can take _____ every thought.

3. Make every thought _____ to Christ.

4. You can demolish _____ and _____ _____that set themselves up against the _____ of God.

In summary, with God's help you are enabled to

- Use spiritual weapons such as the Bible and prayer.
- Challenge any argument that you know contradicts God's truth.
- Refuse to tolerate idle thoughts that could lead to improper action.

➤ How will you use the Bible and prayer in the midst of temptation?

➤ How will you confront ideas that contradict God's truth concerning temptation?

≫ How will you replace idle thoughts before they become temptations?

Whenever possible, we should avoid situations in which you know you will be tempted: certain restaurants and aisles in grocery stores, certain people and entertainment attractions, certain stores and any other place or occasion you know will tempt you. Proverbs 4:14-16 deals with another type of evil situation.

≫ Write Proverbs 4:14-16 in your own words to reinforce this strategy for dealing with temptation.

Another way to avoid temptation is through the truth God gives you. He reveals this truth to you in His Word. God has told you the truth: You can resist temptation.

 Father God, help me to resist temptation today and win because of Your truth in my life.

Lord, help me to avoid the ways of evil men. Turn me away and lead me down Your paths of righteousness.

## DAY 4: *Analyzing and Understanding Temptation*

Tempting thoughts pass through our minds on a regular basis. Dwelling on those thoughts and letting the mind window-shop as it considers them, opens the door to allow us to walk into sin.

≫ What is the primary source of your temptations?

James 1:13-15 has some answers about temptation.

➤ Does God tempt you?

➤ What is the root cause of temptation?

➤ When evil desires grow strong, what results?

➤ What does sin bring into your life?

➤ After reading 1 John 2:15,16, list the three ways temptation plays on your weak nature. (If possible, read this passage in three different translations.)

  1.

  2.

  3.

Temptation is complex, but you can understand it. Temptation plays on your desires, your lusts. It appeals to your passions, your possessions and your pride.

Remember that God doesn't tempt you; He wants to help you. Evil desires are not the same as sin. Left unchecked, evil desires combined with temptation help you decide to sin. In life, sin is always a horrible choice. Sin strangles your spiritual life, choking your relationship with God.

➤ The *King James Version* refers to the three ways of temptation as "the lust of the flesh, and the lust of the eyes, and the pride of life." In relationship to your commitments to First Place, how are you tempted in each of these categories (for example overeating, failure to spend time in Bible Study and prayer, lack of concern for the commitments)? Also record any other area in your life that may bring temptation.

➤ Lust of the flesh

➤ Lust of the eyes

➤ Pride of life

Satan can take things that look good, taste good and feel good and turn them into sinful desires. When facing temptation today, use the promise in Deuteronomy 33:25-27 to find strength.

When sin does enter, you can confess that sin and return to full fellowship with God (see 1 John 1:9). It is much better, though, to avoid sin from the beginning. A problem clearly defined is a problem half solved.

➤ How can the principle of God's provision for a way of escape from temptation and sin help you handle sin more effectively the next time you face temptation?

 Lord God, thank You for helping me to understand temptation and know that You will provide a means of escape.

Father, reveal Your plan for my life. Let me know Your will so that I can follow it and live my life with joy in a closer relationship with You.

# DAY 5: Overcoming Temptation

When temptation comes, you are without excuse. God has set limits on both the tempter and the temptation. God's unlimited power is available for you to use. Your strength may be small, but you can trade your weakness for His strength.

Isaiah 40:29-31 gives powerful hope to those who grow weary of temptation.

≫ God gives _____ to the weary.

≫ God _____ the power of the weak.

≫ What are the four promises for those whose hope is in the Lord?

1.

2.

3.

4.

What power is contained in this passage! What a hope you have in God. What a promise He gives to you. Memorize this verse and use it whenever you feel too tired and weary to keep up your commitments. Let God give you the strength to go on. Let Him take over and breathe life into your weary body.

Read 2 Corinthians 12:9,10 to see what Paul learned about his weaknesses.

≫ Based on these verses, how should you feel about areas of weakness in your life?

≫ What did Paul mean when he said, "I will boast all the more gladly about my weaknesses" (v. 9)?

God promises to make you strong when you are weak. Resisting temptation and relying on God is a testimony and witness to others about your relationship with God. His grace *is* sufficient for you and His power *is* perfect for you. J. B. Phillips translated this passage in 2 Corinthians 12 this way:

> My grace is enough for you: for where there is weakness, my power is shown the more completely." Therefore, I have cheerfully made up my mind to be proud of my weaknesses, because they mean a deeper experience of the power of Christ. I can even enjoy weaknesses, insults, privations, persecutions and difficulties for Christ's sake. For my very weakness makes me strong in him (vv. 9,10).

Although you are weak and vulnerable, God is strong. God will make you aware of His strength working in you. He will teach you to deal with temptation in a way that shows the world that Jesus is living in and working through your life.

Romans 8:1,2 is another wonderful promise for those who are in Christ Jesus.

➳ Rewrite this promise in your own words

 Heavenly Father, teach me Your way to deal with temptation, so the world will know You through Your work in my life.

Christ Jesus, thank You for giving me the law of the Spirit of life to set me free from the law of sin and death.

# DAY 6: *Reflections*

In this week's study you have come to understand temptation and how to overcome it through the grace of God. As you focus on the memory verse this week, ask God how you can put this verse to work in your life.

Memorizing and sharing verses with others gives you the opportunity to share important biblical truths. Think of ways you can give testimony of God's grace in helping you to resist temptation.

With God so intimately involved in your life, He is aware of everything that goes on in it. He knows your weaknesses and provides you a defense against those weaknesses through His powerful Word. Meditate on God's Word and use it in times of stress and temptation, just as Jesus used His Father's Word to defeat Satan in the wilderness. You will be more than a conqueror through Christ Jesus.

Don't wait until you are in the middle of an attack to seek God's guidance. Instead, hide God's Word in your heart in preparation for battle. God's truth sets you free to live. Commit to memory John 8:32. When you know the truth, you will be free from the worries of this world and the sin that entangles you.

Beth Moore devoted a chapter in *Praying God's Word* to just about every stronghold or worldly sin that might come into your life. The chapter on "Overcoming the Enemy" gives a number of verses to memorize and use in prayer time.[1] Remember that "your enemy the devil prowls around like a roaring lion, looking for someone to devour" (1 Peter 5:8). However, you can "resist him, standing firm in the faith" (1 Peter 5:9).

Prayer using Scripture as its focus will help to keep you on course. The following are adapted from chapter 14 of *Praying God's Word*.

Though my enemy plots evil against me and devises wicked schemes, he will not succeed if I am walking with You, O God. You will make him turn his back when You aim at him with drawn bow. Be exalted, O Lord, in Your strength! I will sing and praise Your might! (see Psalm 21:11-13).

Father, I pray that You will cause no weapon forged against me to prevail. Enable me to refute the tongue of my accuser. Thank You for giving this heritage to Your servants (see Isaiah 54:17).

Father, please help me always to know You are near and not to be anxious about anything, but in everything, by prayer and petition, with thanksgiving, to present my requests to You. And when I do, Your peace, which transcends all understanding, will guard my heart and mind in Christ Jesus (see Philippians 4:5-7).[2]

# DAY 7: *Reflections*

As you focus this week on overcoming temptation, think of ways you can prepare yourself for temptations in situations you can't avoid. Stay in tune with God, and have your armor ready for the battle.

When you fill your mind with God's Word, you renew your mind. It guards you against becoming the victim of temptation and protects you from the lures of the world. The temptations and lures will still be there, but you will have the power for victory.

Proverbs 2:7-11 describes the power God offers you and all the protection you need to fight your battles. Memorize verses 10 and 11 of this passage to remind you of the results of godly wisdom. You can apply these two verses to the choices you are making about your physical life.

Work with your flip chart this week, listen to your cassette, and repeat the memory verse from Zechariah 4:6. The Holy Spirit is with you and will guide you and give you victory.

As you apply the principles of Scripture memory from last week, thank God for giving you the opportunity to learn more about His Word and His plan for your life.

My Father, please help me to be on my guard, to stand firm in the faith, to be a person of courage, to be strong and to do everything in love (see 1 Corinthians 16:13).

My faithful Father, help me to have absolute assurance that I am a child of God because the whole world system is presently under the control of the evil one (see 1 John 5:19).

Father God, You promised victory, not by might or by power, but by Your Spirit. Let Your Spirit dwell in me so that I might experience Your victory in my life (see Zechariah 4:6).

Notes
1. Beth Moore, *Praying God's Word* (Nashville, TN: Broadman and Holman, 2000), pp. 301-333.
2. Ibid., pp. 317, 325, 328.

# GROUP PRAYER REQUESTS   TODAY'S DATE:_____

| NAME | REQUEST | RESULTS |
|------|---------|---------|
|      |         |         |
|      |         |         |
|      |         |         |
|      |         |         |
|      |         |         |
|      |         |         |
|      |         |         |
|      |         |         |
|      |         |         |
|      |         |         |
|      |         |         |
|      |         |         |
|      |         |         |

# HANDLING GUILT

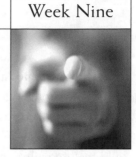

## MEMORY VERSE

*Therefore, there is now no condemnation*
*for those who are in Christ Jesus.*

Romans 8:1

Momentary failures mix with ongoing success as you work to change areas of your life. As you try to make changes, don't be devastated if you lose a few battles on your way to victory. In a weak moment you may be tempted; if you indulge, you'll probably feel guilty.

In this week's study, you'll learn more about guilt. You'll learn about the type of guilt on which the Bible focuses. You'll also learn about guilty feelings common to the Christian life. In addition, you'll examine principles for living in spiritual victory. Increasing victory will result in less guilt in your life.

## DAY 1: *God's Incredible Provision*

Reading passages in the Bible that contain the word "guilt" reveals this truth: Everyone stands guilty before God. Romans 3:23 provides God's bottom-line assessment about the source of this guilt—our sin.

➤ Rewrite Romans 3:23 in your own words.

Why do people feel guilty? The Bible's answer? Because we *are* guilty. In the same way, a sick person could ask "Why am I running a fever?" A doctor could respond "Because you *are* sick." Fever is a symptom of illness; guilty feelings are symptoms of the shame of sin.

≫ According to Psalm 38:4, how does guilt feel?

Guilt becomes a heavy, overwhelming load. Some people, however, don't seem to feel guilty about their relationship with God. Remember, a person can be critically ill without experiencing symptoms of illness. In the same way, someone can be spiritually guilty before God without actually feeling guilty. In either case, physical illness or spiritual guilt, feelings do not change the facts.

≫ With physical illness, why is it dangerous to treat the symptoms rather than deal with the disease?

Many contemporary self-help solutions to life's problems offer people emotional aspirin when what is really need is spiritual surgery. God identifies the basic problem and offers a true solution.

≫ Read each of the following verses; then list the key words or phrases that explain God's attitude toward you and the way He responds to you.

| Scriptures | Key Words and Phrases |
|---|---|
| Psalm 32:5 | |
| Psalm 51:1,2 | |
| Psalm 86:5 | |
| Psalm 130:3,4 | |
| Psalm 130:7,8 | |

God loves you, even when you sin, and He will forgive your sins when you confess them.

➻ Rewrite 1 John 1:9 in your own words.

Your sins left you guilty before God. Christ died to pay your spiritual debt. Accept the forgiveness He made available to you. If you have not invited Jesus Christ to be the Lord of your life, why not deal with it right now? Pray and confess your sin to God. Open your life to God. If He is the Lord of your life, pray for forgiveness of sin and ask Him to show you the way He wants you to go.

Heavenly Father, I come to You seeking forgiveness for my sin and ask that You take away my guilt and pain and let me serve You.

Father, I seek Your unfailing love and full redemption from all my sin.

## DAY 2: *No Condemnation in Jesus Christ*

In your physical life, fever indicates disease exists so that you can seek treatment. In our spiritual life, guilty feelings indicate a broken relationship with God exists so that you can seek redemption. These symptoms, fever or guilt, prompt you to take action.

➻ According to John 16:8, what is the source of feelings of guilt?

Conviction, an awareness of your separation from God, prompts you to reach out to God. While the Holy Spirit works to convict people of sin, Christians must always remember that because of Jesus Christ, you are not guilty of sin. Christ paid for your sins on the cross. Is it ever appropriate for Christians to feel guilty? The key word is "feel." You should feel remorse when you don't live up to your potential in Christ. You should feel disappointed when you don't draw fully on the Holy Spirit's power to resist temptation. You should not, however, allow feelings of guilt to overwhelm you and hinder your ability to move on in life.

The good news is that God receives you as His own child when you respond in faith to Him. God takes Christ's death on the cross and credits it as the punishment for your sins. Your debt is paid. You are forgiven. No longer do you have reason to feel guilty.

How do you as a Christian handle guilt? Here are two principles to guide you.

- When you sin, you must immediately confess that sin to God, receive His cleansing and restore the intimacy of your relationship with God.
- You must learn from your experience with sin and trust the Holy Spirit to help you avoid that sin in the future.

➣ What is Satan called in Revelation 12:10?

In your spiritual battle, Satan enjoys playing the role of the accuser. He delights in telling you, "You feel guilty because you are guilty. You failed this time. You will always fail."

Hebrews 10:17 tells you how God views your sins since you've become a Christian.

➣ According to this verse, once I became a Christian, God remembers

my _____ and _____ no more.

➣ According to Psalm 103:12, what does God do with your sin once you confess it to Him?

How far *is* the east from the west? That's how far God removes your sin. He forgives totally. He chooses not to remember your sin.

≫ What if you continue to struggle with guilt after you become a Christian? Reread the memory verse, Romans 8:1, then write the verse.

≫ What does this verse mean to you?

As a Christian you stand cleansed before God. No condemnation remains. God has forgiven you. You live now as His child. Any guilt or condemnation you feel does not come from God.

Lord Jesus, thank You for the price You paid so that I can stand before You without guilt.

Heavenly Father, I praise Your name because You made it possible for me to enjoy peace in my relationship with You. I give You praise because in Christ there is no condemnation.

# DAY 3: *The Life-Transforming Gospel*

For the first 11 chapters of Romans, Paul focused on God's glorious plan of salvation. His argument reached its culmination in Romans 12:1.

≫ Rewrite this verse in your own words.

The *good news*, or *gospel*, should transform the way you live. In the chart below, read each basic principle listed on the left. These principles are drawn from the good news of your relationship with Christ. Then write a statement on the right side of the chart describing a practical way you can use the principle in your daily life.

| Positive Truths of the Gospel | How I Can Apply Them in My Life |
|---|---|
| I am a valuable person. Christ was willing to die on the cross for me. | |
| I am forgiven. My debt of sin has been fully paid by Jesus Christ. | |
| God knows every sin I have committed or ever will commit and still loves me. | |
| God now lives in my life. I can live with His spiritual power. | |

The key to living the Christian life with victory is the Holy Spirit. Through the Holy Spirit, God works in your life. Without the Spirit's power, you doom yourself to frustration and perpetual cycles of failure and guilt. With the Spirit, you can learn to live in fullness.

➤ In Ephesians 5:18, Paul contrasted being filled with the Spirit and being drunk with wine. Why do you think he used this contrast?

Americans have become aware of the devastating consequences that result when people operate their cars while DUI (driving under the influence of alcohol). No image could provide a more striking negative contrast to the Holy Spirit and the positive influence He brings to people's lives. When God's Spirit lives in you, His influence can be seen; His positive influence impacts all you do.

Father God, help me to live my life each day with the awareness of what Jesus Christ did for me.

Lord, allow my relationship with You to transform my attitudes and my habits.

## DAY 4: *The Struggle with Sin*

The Christian life is based on grand truths about God's love, forgiveness and power. When we become Christians, we want to live a life that glorifies God. We want to make changes that will please Him. But will these changes be automatic and effortless? Even great Christians like the apostle Paul struggled with sin, as we read in Romans 7:15.

➣ How did Paul describe his actions?

How readily you can identify with Paul! You can say "The good things I want to do, I don't do." This creates real frustration.

➣ In Romans 7:18, what more did Paul say about his struggle with sin?

Plenty of desire, but little follow-through—that's another problem that plagues everyone. You know what you want to do—the right thing. Yet you still struggle to do it!

➣ In Romans 7:24, Paul expressed his frustration with sin. How was Paul feeling about his sin and what was his plea?

➤ Who rescued him, according to Romans 7:25a?

There will be times when you fail. Along the way, you'll struggle. But you don't need to feel helpless or trapped. You simply need to learn how to live in the power of His Spirit. Galatians 5:25 describes the relationship you are to maintain with the Holy Spirit.

➤ Since we_____ by the Spirit, let us _____
_____with the Spirit.

Lord God, thank You that through Jesus Christ I can live in victory over sin.

Father, let Your Holy Spirit fill my life to control and empower me to always live under Your influence.

## DAY 5: *The Holy Spirit in You*

Because God's Holy Spirit lives in you, you can reject Satan's lies. You can affirm the truth: In Christ, you are not guilty. Because of Christ, you can live in power. Through the Holy Spirit, you can break the cycle of sin, failure and guilt.

To live with spiritual victory and avoid the cycles of failure and guilt, we must learn how God works in our lives through the Holy Spirit.

➤ As you read the verses in the following chart, what ideas are common in all of these verses? Write a sentence in the right-hand column that expresses the central truth these verses reveal about the Christian and the Holy Spirit.

| Scriptures | Truths About the Holy Spirit |
|---|---|
| Romans 8:9 | |
| 1 Corinthians 3:16 | |
| 1 John 4:13 | |

The Bible clearly states that if the Holy Spirit is not living in you, you are not a Christian. Christianity is not a religion; it is a relationship with God. God relates to you through His Holy Spirit living in you. It is through God's Holy Spirit that you have spiritual power to change the way you live.

➤ Each of the following verses tells something the Holy Spirit wants to do in your life. Match the following principles with the verses from which they are drawn:

_____ 1. Helps me resist the desires of my sinful nature.      a.  Galatians 5:22,23

_____ 2. Helps me live with power, love and discipline.      b.  Ephesians 3:16

_____ 3. Gives me spiritual power in my inner being.      c.  Galatians 5:16

_____ 4. Produces positive character traits in my life.      d.  2 Timothy 1:7

Heavenly Father, thank You for the Holy Spirit's work in me. Let the Holy Spirit broaden Your influence in my life.

Christ Jesus, help me to learn to live in victory through the power of the Holy Spirit.

# DAY 6: *Reflections*

In this week's study you have learned about God's incredible provision to help you handle guilt feelings you develop when you indulge in unacceptable behavior. God loves you even when you sin, and will forgive your sins when you confess them.

King David confessed his sins to God and asked for forgiveness. His words are found in many of the psalms. You may feel completely helpless as David did on several occasions, but learn these words David prayed so that you can pour out your heart to God and seek forgiveness.

Memorize some of the verses you studied this week, and you will have a powerful weapon to help you overcome the stronghold of guilt. Yes, guilt can be a stronghold when it takes over your life and keeps you from having fellowship with God.

Charles Stanley said, "If you assume that because you have failed God once—or even more than once—in the past, He will never use you in the future, you're limiting God."[1] God didn't send His Son into the world to condemn it but so that the world might be saved through Him. Refuse to accept the guilt of your past sins and look ahead to the forgiveness that is yours as a child of God.

Remember that God's truth, His Word, will set you free. The following prayers are based on verses from the book of Psalms. Memorize the verses and use them in your prayer time.

Heavenly Father, create in me a pure heart and renew a steadfast spirit within me. Do not cast me from Your presence or take Your Holy Spirit from me. Restore to me the joy of Your salvation and grant me a willing spirit to sustain me (see Psalm 51:10-12).

You are forgiving and good, O Lord. Your love abounds to all who call to You. Hear my prayer, and listen to my cry for mercy. In the day of my trouble I will call to You, for You will answer me (see Psalm 86:5-7).

Father, if You kept a record of sins, O Lord, who could stand? But with You there is forgiveness; therefore You are feared (see Psalm 130:3,4).

# DAY 7: *Reflections*

As you focus this week on overcoming feelings of guilt, think of ways you can overcome temptations and avoid guilt feelings. Stay in tune with God, and have your armor ready for the battle.

Use the principles of Scripture memory from Week Seven and find verses that will help you when you yield to temptation and experience feelings of guilt. The Holy Spirit through God's Word will help you live in power, love and self-discipline.

As a Christian, you can have a deep, personal relationship with God through His Holy Spirit living in you. To live by the Spirit, you must learn to keep in step with the Spirit, following His leadership in your life. The Holy Spirit doesn't force you to yield to His control. Ask the Holy Spirit to empower your life through God's Word.

As you read God's Word, underline, highlight or write in your journal significant Scriptures. Commit them to memory to have when you are faced with feelings of guilt.

The following prayers may help get you started:

Father God, You have told me to live by the Spirit so that I will not gratify the desires of my sinful nature. Help me, Father, to live by Your Spirit that You gave me (see Galatians 5:16).

Father God, give me strength so that I will not grieve the Holy Spirit by whom I was sealed for the day of redemption (see Ephesians 4:30).

My faithful Father, out of Your glorious riches strengthen me with power through Your Spirit in my innermost being (see Ephesians 3:16).

Father God, I believe Your Word when You said there is no condemnation for those who are in Christ Jesus. Thank You for that promise (see Romans 8:1).

Note
1. Charles Stanley, *In Touch with God* (Nashville, TN: Thomas Nelson, 1997), p. 41.

# GROUP PRAYER REQUESTS  TODAY'S DATE:_____

| NAME | REQUEST | RESULTS |
|------|---------|---------|
|      |         |         |
|      |         |         |
|      |         |         |
|      |         |         |
|      |         |         |
|      |         |         |
|      |         |         |
|      |         |         |
|      |         |         |
|      |         |         |
|      |         |         |
|      |         |         |
|      |         |         |

# KNOWING GOD

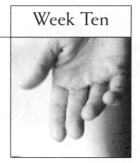

*Those who know your name will trust in you,*
*for you, LORD, have never forsaken*
*those who seek you.*
Psalm 9:10

During Old Testament times, a person's name often gave an indication of his character or some personal quality. In the Bible, there are several names for God. Each name reveals a different aspect of His character. It's similar to the way we use different names according to our roles in life. One woman may be called mother, sister, daughter, wife, nurse, aunt, friend, etc. The name someone uses reveals something about her relationship to that person.

One name cannot encompass God's greatness. One name imposes limitations on God. If all the universe cannot contain God, how can one name ever hope to describe Him? In this week's study, you'll learn how each of God's names shows you a specific way to relate to Him and how that relationship meets a particular need in your life.

## DAY 1: *Elohim, the Source of All Creation*

In the first verse of the Bible, Genesis 1:1 the word "God" is translated from the Hebrew word *Elohim*. When this word is used for God, it refers to Him as creator of all things. It attempts to describe His omnipotence and His sovereignty. For us, it means God is the source—all we have comes from Him.

➤ According to James 1:17, God is the source of every good and perfect gift. List several good gifts God has given you.

➤ God gave you a perfect gift. Romans 8:32 says that gift is

_____.

If God did nothing more than give you Jesus, that would be enough—far more than you could ever dream possible. But God continues to give you good gifts.

➤ Isaiah 40:28 describes another gift God continues to give you. What is it?

Not only did God create the world, He also created each one of us. As your creator, He knows everything about you, including your needs. God is intimately involved in the world He created. God wants to be intimately involved in your life.

Matthew 6:8 tells the depth of God's understanding of your life.

➤ How well does God know your needs?

Isn't that a wonderful thought? Before you even begin to pray, God knows your needs. Despite knowing this, there are times when you may wonder if God can deal with all the problems you face.

In Jeremiah 32:27, God responds to someone who questioned His strength.

➤ What was the question?

➤ The answer can be found in Jeremiah 32:17. What *is* the answer?

God, the creator of all things, points to the world He made and says, "I have enough power to create all this! Don't you think I have enough power for the things you face in your life?" The God of creative power is the God who loves you. Nothing you ever face in life is too difficult for Him—not even your strongholds in healthy living.

When you have a need in your life, whether it is physical, emotional or spiritual, remember that nothing is too difficult for God. Turn to Him as your God, *Elohim*, the source of all creation.

Heavenly Father, I come to You as the creator of the universe, thanking You for Your great gifts of life and of the Holy Spirit through Your son, Jesus Christ.

Elohim, nothing is too difficult for You, and I come to You with all my burdens and cares because I know You will take care of me. Thank You for Your love.

## DAY 2: *Jehovah, God Who Is Always There; El Roi, God Who Sees*

These two names, *Jehovah* and *El Roi*, for God fit together like a hand in a glove. Jehovah is the most frequently used name for God in the modern translation of the Bible. It speaks of God's being, His essence. The name "Jehovah" reminds us that God is, was and always will be. He is the omnipresent God. El Roi is ever watchful, aware of all circumstances that affect your life. Others may be unaware of the small victories in your life, but your El Roi knows and cares about those small successes as well as the big ones.

Since Jehovah is always there, then El Roi is aware of everything that happens in your life. Exodus 3:13,14 describes when Moses asked Jehovah what to say if the Israelites asked His name.

➤ What did God tell Moses to call Him?

≫ What do you think God wanted to communicate by calling Himself "I Am"?

Bible scholars and students have puzzled for years over God's response to Moses. At the very least, God wanted Moses, and you, to understand that He has always existed in the past and will exist in the future. God is not locked in time; He stands outside time. As a result, God has no limitation in time or space.

Since God has no limitations, He is aware of everything that happens in your life. You do many things in your life that no one sees or notices, but God knows.

≫ Joshua 1:8—How does God bless you when you continue to meditate on His Word?

≫ Matthew 6:6—How have you experienced God's reward when you pray in private?

≫ Galatians 6:9—What will you ultimately receive when you struggle yet persevere?

These are great promises from our Jehovah, who can do anything, and El Roi, who sees everything. Since God is not limited in any way, He is constantly available to you.

≫ What does Psalm 139:7-10 tell you about God's presence in your life?




≫ What is the promise found in Hebrews 13:5b?




≫ What practical effect should this promise have on the way you live?




≫ How does Isaiah 26:4 describe God?




As a Christian, you live with God's promise that He is constantly with you. Wherever you are, whatever you do, God is there and sees all that you do. God is your eternal rock. When you need consistency and stability in your life, turn to your Jehovah who loves you. When you feel no one loves or appreciates all that you do, turn to your El Roi, the One who sees and knows what you do. God is, was and always will be.

 Jehovah, thank You for always being present in my time of trouble and need.

El Roi, I praise Your name because You are the One who knows me as I am and sees all that I do and forgives me when I fail.

# DAY 3: *Jehovah-Jireh, God Who Provides*

The early Israelites often combined the name of God with other words to more accurately describe characteristics of God. He is more than Jehovah, the self-existent one. God is *Jehovah-Jireh*, which means "the Lord will provide."

The Old Testament tells the story of Abraham and his son, Isaac, going to Mount Moriah to offer a sacrifice to God in Genesis 22:1-19.

➤ When Isaac asked his father about a lamb for the sacrifice, what was Abraham's reply?

➤ What event is being foreshadowed in Genesis 22:8?

➤ How did God provide for Abraham?

In the same way God provided for Abraham and Isaac, so God continues to provide for you. God did provide a lamb for you—Jesus Christ, the Lamb of God who takes away the sin of the world.

➤ What is the promise found in Philippians 4:19?

➤ What do you need to do, according to Luke 11:9,10?

➥ What does Hebrews 4:16 say about approaching God?

God is not reluctant to meet your needs. Although the timing isn't always clear and you may often wonder about the nature of His provision, in time you can always acknowledge that God did provide for you.

➥ Describe a time when God provided for you in a special way.

If you need strength to resist temptation or if you need encouragement to go on, turn to Jehovah-Jireh. Seek Him, and you will find mercy. Seek Him, and you will find grace. Seek Him, and Jehovah-Jireh will provide.

Jehovah-Jireh, I praise Your name and give thanks to You who provides for my needs and cares for me like no other.

Lord, You have promised to meet all my needs in every situation. I claim that promise and look to You for provision of my mental, spiritual, physical and emotional needs.

## DAY 4: *Jehovah-Shalom, God Our Peace; Jehovah-Rohi, God Our Shepherd*

Through the name *Jehovah-Shalom*, God reveals Himself as the Lord of peace. We never truly appreciate nor long for peace until we find ourselves in a desperate situation. Then we cry out for peace; our sanity depends on it. Thank God, He is our peace.

Jehovah-Rohi is the name for God the shepherd, who brings peace and comfort to the hearts of believers everywhere. The shepherd will lead you to safety and protect you from danger. In that safety you can feel the peace that comes only from knowing and following the shepherd.

➥ What is Jesus called in John 10:11 and what will He do for you?

Read and then answer the following questions:

➤ According to John 10:27, how are you learning to hear His voice?

➤ How well are you following Jesus?

➤ According to Isaiah 26:3, what is the key to having a sense of peace in every situation?

➤ According to Philippians 4:6,7, how is it possible to live and not worry?

➤ How should you make your requests known to God?

➤ Describe a time that you have experienced the peace of God that "transcends all understanding."

As your good shepherd, Jesus provides for your needs.

➤ According to 1 Peter 2:2, what is spiritual milk and what does it do in your life?

➤ In Psalm 23:4, why should you "fear no evil"?

When you feel the need for someone to care for you or when you need guidance and direction, turn to Jehovah-Rohi, your good shepherd, who will lead you in paths of righteousness, and to Jehovah-Shalom who will say to your heart, "Peace; be still."

Jehovah-Shalom, thank You for the peace that passes all understanding, even in the midst of turmoil in my life.

Jehovah-Rohi, lead me and guide me as the shepherd leads His sheep through the deep valleys of death or beside the cool waters. Lead me to safety and protect me from danger.

## DAY 5: _Jehovah-Sabaoth, God Who Delivers Us_

When the children of Israel needed deliverance from hopeless situations, they came to know God as _Jehovah-Sabaoth_. The word "sabaoth" refers to a mass of people or things—an army, for example. When you call to God as your Jehovah-Sabaoth, you can see Him as a mighty army that confronts your needs and gives you victory.

➤ After you read each of the following verses, write down what that verse says about the God who delivers you.

Psalm 18:2

Psalm 70:5


Psalm 144:2


As you face challenges in life, Jehovah-Sabaoth will be your help, your rock, your stronghold—everything you will ever need to help in fighting the battles against your enemy.

> ➤ After you read Psalm 31:2; 2 Timothy 4:18 and 2 Peter 2:9, summarize the common ideas in all three verses and how they relate to your efforts in First Place.


A five-year-old child was lying in a sterile hospital bed in isolation, diagnosed with meningitis. No visitors were allowed inside the room, so her grandmother sat outside the door and spoke to the child through an intercom system. The grandmother repeated the words of Psalm 27:1 over and over to the small, sobbing child. Slowly the child ceased her cries and fell asleep. All night the grandmother kept her vigil, praying for and singing to the child. She repeated several times, "Don't be afraid. God is your light. He is your stronghold. He's taking care of you." The next morning, after another painful spinal tap, the doctors could find no traces of the meningitis. The child grew in the goodness of the Lord and never forgot those words of strength and comfort prayed by a loving grandmother. Years later as an adult, she had opportunity to again recall those words when faced with cancer. She knew that she had nothing to fear with God as her light and salvation, her stronghold who could deliver her from any attack.

✺ Read Psalm 27:1-3. What does verse 1 tell you about Jehovah-Sabaoth?

"The Lord is _____

_____."

"The Lord is _____

_____."

Summarize verses 2 and 3.


God promises to rescue you from situations in life that threaten to overwhelm you. You have someone to whom you can turn in the midst of fear and struggles. When from a human perspective you feel trapped, turn to your Jehovah-Sabaoth and He will rescue you.

Heavenly Father, thank You for being the stronghold in my life and delivering me from those things that threaten me.

Jehovah-Sabaoth, be my deliverer. Help me in time of trouble and give me comfort when all around me is falling apart.


# DAY 6: *Reflections*

In this week's study you have learned about the many names of God that describe His many functions in your life. He is a God who knows you, sees you, loves you, forgives you, leads you, delivers you, gives you peace and is the creator of all things. What an incredible provision He makes for you in time of struggle, when you feel trapped.

No matter what name you give Him, He is still the God of the way, the truth and the light. His truths are everlasting. Bible study shows you verses to use in any situation at any time in your life. If the verses are hidden in your heart, you will never be without them. Though your Bible be taken away and destroyed, the Word cannot be taken from your heart.

Review the various days of reflection and the methods discussed to help you memorize Scripture. If you have followed along and memorized the memory verse for each week, you now have 10 powerful weapons to use for your everyday victories.

We are an ordinary people in an ordinary world with an extraordinary God. Allow Him to give you victory through His Word, and He will teach you to trust Him completely.

 Heavenly Father, I know my help comes from You, who made heaven and earth. You will not allow my foot to slip; You will not slumber (see Psalm 121:2,3).

Jehovah, You are my refuge and my fortress. O my God, in You I will trust. You will save me from the fowler's snare and from the deadly pestilence. You shall cover me with Your feathers, and under Your wings I shall take refuge. Your faithfulness shall be my shield and rampart (see Psalm 91:2-4).

## DAY 7: *Reflections*

Congratulations! You've completed the course!

As you come to the end of this study, focus on the many names and attributes of God. Use the principles of Scripture memory to find verses that will help you to have an even better understanding of the names of God.

In the Old Testament, the people of God knew Him only through His many names. They depended on the prophets to lead them and give them instructions from God. In the New Testament, God sent the Holy Spirit through His Son, Jesus Christ, to teach and guide us.

Although the session has ended, you can continue with your commitments to the program in your daily life. Keep studying the Bible daily, memorizing Scripture and praying. If you haven't started a prayer journal, it's not too late to begin one now and add to it daily. What you have learned these past 10 weeks can be used to gain those everyday victories that give you the strength to carry on to the next day.

Your First Place leaders wish you the very best in continuing the efforts begun 10 weeks ago. Even if you didn't reach your goal for the session, you are not a failure. You simply are not as far along as you had hoped to be. God is faithful and will continue to work in your life if you give Him control. May God richly bless you in the coming weeks and we hope you continue the First Place Bible studies.

Father God, You are the vine, and I am one of the branches. If I remain in You and You in me, I will bear much fruit, because without You, I can do nothing (see John 15:5).

Father God, I know You chose me and appointed me to go and bear fruit—fruit that will last. Then You, O Father, will give me whatever I ask in Your name (see John 15:16).

Heavenly Father, You promised to instruct me and teach me in the way I should go; You will then guide me with Your eye (see Psalm 32:8).

Father God, You have said those who know Your name will trust in You, for You, Lord, have never forsaken those who seek You (see Psalm 9:10).

# GROUP PRAYER REQUESTS   TODAY'S DATE:_____

| NAME | REQUEST | RESULTS |
|------|---------|---------|
|      |         |         |
|      |         |         |
|      |         |         |
|      |         |         |
|      |         |         |
|      |         |         |
|      |         |         |
|      |         |         |
|      |         |         |
|      |         |         |
|      |         |         |
|      |         |         |
|      |         |         |

# CONVENIENCE FOODS:
## *Making the Most of Your Time*

Does life have you on the go? Of course it does! Our fast-paced lives require us to cook and eat on the run. Fortunately grocery store aisles are filled with convenience foods of all types—frozen dinners, canned soups, ready-to-eat cereals—and they come in all types of packages—jars, cans, bottles, boxes and bags. These foods save time in our busy lives, but they can also be high in calories, fat, cholesterol, added sugars and sodium.

Don't let busyness become a roadblock to achieving and maintaining a healthy weight and following a nutritious eating plan. The keys to healthy nutrition are balance, moderation and variety, even in convenience foods.

## READING LABELS

The most popular trend in convenience foods over the last several years is the introduction of *low-fat foods*. Low-fat versions of our favorite foods are everywhere. Recently one shopper was quoted as saying: "There's low-fat, no fat, fat-free, nonfat and 95 percent fat-free- I spent half the morning at the grocery store just looking at brownie labels!" You may feel the same way. You would think with all the low-fat foods available, Americans would be losing pounds by the truckload. However, surveys show that Americans are gaining more weight than ever. There's one important thing to keep in mind: *Low fat doesn't necessarily mean low calorie!*

| Product | Calories | Product | Calories |
|---|---|---|---|
| Chocolate cream-filled cookie | 53 | Fat-free version | 55 |
| Fig bar | 60 | Fat-free version | 70 |
| Granola cereal | 130 | Reduced-fat version | 110 |
| Breakfast bar | 120 | Reduced-fat version | 120 |
| 3-ounce bagel | 150 | Today's bigger version | 400 |

Next time you shop, compare the calories on the low-fat foods you buy with the regular versions. Is there really a difference? Compare serving sizes too. Sometimes the difference in calories is actually due to the smaller size!

# Choosing Healthy Convenience Foods

Dinners and single-item foods can fit into your daily balance of calories, fat, cholesterol, sodium, fiber and sugar. Use these healthful guidelines to help you choose healthier convenience foods.

| Look for Foods | Look for Clues on the Food Label | Know Your Daily Goal |
|---|---|---|
| Low in fat | 3 g or less per serving | 30% or less of total calories |
| Low in saturated fat | 1 g or less per serving | less than 10% of total calories |
| Low in cholesterol | 60 mg or less per serving | less than 300 mg |
| Low in sodium | less than 400 mg per serving | less than 2400 mg |
| High in fiber | 2.5 g or more per serving | 25-30 g |
| High in nutrients | 10% or more of the Reference Daily Intake (RDI)[1] for one or more of the following: vitamin A, vitamin C, iron, calcium, protein and fiber | 100% of the RDI |

1. Reference Daily Intake (RDI) is a new term that replaces U.S. Recommended Daily Allowance (RDA). The percentages that a food contributes to the RDI for these nutrients are listed on the food label.

When choosing frozen dinners or entrees, use the following guidelines:

- Choose dinners that have less than 400 calories, 15 grams of fat, 5 grams of saturated fat and 800 milligrams of sodium.

- Choose entrees with less than 300 calories, 10 grams of fat and 4 grams of saturated fat.

## Using Convenience Foods

- Compare food labels when shopping for convenience foods. Choose the food with the lowest saturated fat, cholesterol and sodium.

- When cooking packaged foods, such as instant noodles or macaroni and cheese, lower the fat and calories by using less butter or margarine than the directions call for. Use half of the seasoning packet, or use your own seasonings, to lower the sodium content. Add your own fresh or frozen vegetables to add fiber, vitamins and minerals.

- When buying canned meat such as chicken, tuna or salmon, choose water-packed varieties instead of oil-packed.

- Choose breakfast cereals with terms such as "high fiber," "whole grain" or "bran" on the label. Cereals that are high in fiber (>2.5 grams per serving) and low in added sugar are good choices.

- Canned or frozen fruits and vegetables are good choices, but watch out for sodium and added fats. Rinse vegetables, beans and canned meats with water to reduce the sodium content. Avoid canned and frozen vegetables with high-fat sauces.

- Limit use of frozen dinners and entrees with breaded or fried meats and vegetables.

- Buy prepackaged salads instead of individual ingredients. Buy products with an assortment of lettuce and other fresh vegetables. Be wary of those that come with their own dressings and croutons which are high in fat.

- Increase nutrients by balancing out your meal with a piece of fruit and a low-fat dairy product, such as nonfat milk.

- Prepare your own healthy convenience foods by cooking your own recipes and freezing the leftovers in individual servings. Freezer bags and a variety of plastic containers make it convenient for you to store and reheat your meals.

What types of convenience foods do you most often use? List a few healthy changes you can make when buying, preparing and eating these foods.

| Food | Healthy Change |
|------|----------------|
|      |                |
|      |                |
|      |                |
|      |                |

# GROUP EXERCISE FOR FUN AND FITNESS

Group exercise simply refers to a group of people exercising together under the direction of an instructor. Often the exercises are set to music. The instructor, group members and music all work together to create a fun and beneficial workout. Group exercise classes are offered at fitness clubs, community centers and some workplaces. You can even do group exercise at home with special videotapes. If you want, find a qualified instructor and get your own group together in the neighborhood, at church or at work.

Here's a list of some of the most popular group classes. Which ones do you enjoy?

☐ Aerobic dance (low/high-impact)     ☐ Indoor Cycling
☐ Group calisthenics/flexibility      ☐ Water aerobics
☐ Circuit weight training             ☐ Jazzercise
☐ Boxing-type workouts                ☐ Stepping (low/impact)
☐ Combination of various types        ☐ Other _____

## THE BENEFITS OF GROUP EXERCISE

Check out the following benefits of group exercise. If several of these benefits sound important to you, group exercise may be a good choice.

🍎 It's more fun to exercise with others.

🍎 A well-trained instructor can provide motivation and education.

🍎 The group can be a source of accountability.

🍎 Provides variety for your physical activity routine.

🍎 The music and environment make exercise more enjoyable.

🍎 Can provide a total body workout: aerobics, strength building and stretching.

# FIRST STEPS

## Choosing the Right Instructor

Look for a nationally certified instructor who has the experience and knowledge to provide you with a safe, effective and enjoyable workout. A good instructor will learn your name, make eye contact during the session and put your workout before his or her own. The instructor should have you take your heart rate or teach you how to rate your intensity level. A good teacher will explain the benefits of each exercise, demonstrate how to do the exercise and modify movements for all skill and fitness levels.

## Clothing and Shoes

Usually you don't need any special clothing. Choose clothing that allows you to move freely. It's important that the clothes you choose breathe, allowing sweat to evaporate. Avoid rubber suits and sweatshirts that don't absorb or pull moisture away from the skin. Most important, wear clothing that is comfortable—put fitness ahead of fashion! For dance or step classes, choose an aerobic shoe with good cushioning. Good heel and arch support is important. The shoe should be flexible, provide a broad base of support and have plenty of room for your toes. Running or walking shoes are not a good choice because they don't provide the support you need for side-to-side movements. A high-top shoe might provide more ankle support. Shop for shoes carefully.

## Precautions

Before you reserve your spot in a group class, you need to take a few precautions.

- *If you're a man over 40 or a woman over 50, or if you have underlying health problems, check with your doctor before participating in a vigorous exercise class.*

- Some aerobic dance and step classes are high impact (i.e., a lot of hopping, jumping and jogging). If you're just starting out or you have knee, ankle or back problems, choose classes that are low impact. Some classes can also be difficult if you have poor balance or coordination. Water aerobics might be a better choice.

- The skill and fitness levels needed for various classes differ. Choose a class that's best for you. The class should not fatigue or exhaust you. If you initially find the class difficult to follow, focus on learning the movements before worrying about intensity. Avoid exercising at a higher level of intensity than your body is used to; it's easy to overexert yourself trying to keep up with the class. If you have a hard time keeping up, slow down and take a break when necessary. Remember, you're doing this for your own health and fitness—not to compete with others.

🍎 Learning to maintain proper body alignment and technique helps prevent injuries. Maintain good posture with shoulders back, chest lifted, back straight and pelvis tucked under. Try to stay relaxed and breathe easily. Avoid any movements that are uncomfortable for you or seem to put stress on your joints. Just because an instructor does a movement doesn't mean it's right for you. Talk to your instructor about other movements or stretches you can do instead. Using hand weights can increase the risk of injury in aerobic dance and stepping classes. In stepping classes avoid using benches that are too high—start with a 4- to 6-inch bench and work your way up as your fitness improves.

🍎 Drink plenty of water. Drink at least eight ounces of water 15 minutes before class and continue to drink water every 15 to 20 minutes during class. It's a good idea to keep a water bottle nearby while you exercise.

## COMPONENTS OF A GROUP EXERCISE CLASS

Most classes consist of four or five phases. Each phase has an important purpose for both fitness and safety. These same phases should be a part of any exercise or physical activity you do.

🍎 **Warm-Up Phase**—This prepares the body for more vigorous activity by allowing muscles and joints to loosen up and the heart and lungs to gradually begin delivering more blood andoxygen to the muscles. The warm-up should consist of at least 5 to 10 minutes of light activity and stretching.

🍎 **Aerobic Phase**—This consists of continuous and rhythmic movement designed to improve health and cardiovascular endurance. The aerobic phase should not feel hard and should last 20 to 30 minutes. If the pace is uncomfortable or you're breathing so hard you can't carry on a conversation, *slow down!*

- **Transition Phase**—This short phase of light activity is important when you move from the aerobics phase to the calisthenics and flexibility phase.

- **Calisthenics and Flexibility Phase**—This consists of strengthening and stretching exercises to condition and tone the muscles, improve range of motion and lower the risk of injury.

- **Cooldown Phase**—This allows time for the body to safely transition back to normal activity. It's very important not to stop abruptly following moderate to vigorous activity. The cooldown should consist of at least 5 to 10 minutes of light activity and stretching.

# LETTING OTHERS HELP YOU SUCCEED

It's important to find people who can help you achieve and maintain your goals and then get them involved in providing the support and encouragement you need. Communication is the cornerstone of any relationship. You must tell your partner what you need. Ask him or her to do specific things to help you. Never expect your partner to read your mind. Tell him or her when you need encouragement. Point out (in a positive way!) when you need him or her to respond or treat you differently. Ask frequently what you can do for your partner. Surprise him or her with rewards that show your appreciation. For a partnership to be successful, the relationship must be one where each partner gives a little and takes a little.

## KINDS OF SUPPORT

There are many types of support. Think about the types of support you need and who can best help.

- **Do you need someone to talk to?** It's important to be able to share your feelings and experiences with others. Sometimes all you need is someone to listen. It's important to be able to share both positive and negative aspects of your life.

  With whom can you best share your feelings and experiences?

  Who can help you develop and stick with realistic goals and plans for lifestyle change?

  Who can you turn to when you are struggling or get off track?

- **Do you need someone to participate with you?** It's often easier and more fun to make lifestyle changes when others are involved.

  Would your spouse or a friend go through the program with you?

  Who would be someone to exercise with?

  Will it help if your family makes some changes with you?

🍎 **Do you need someone to provide you with encouragement?** It's easier to make changes when others are encouraging and supporting you. It's easy to get discouraged when you slip up or don't reach your goals as quickly as you would like.

Who can help pick you up when you get down and discouraged?

Who can reward you as you reach your goals?

Who is a good encourager for you?

Sometimes it's important to have constructive criticism. Who would help you stay on your goals and push you when you need it?

Ask others to give you the feedback you need—and be willing to accept what they say. Who is the best person to help you in this way?

🍎 **Do you need someone to help with other aspects of your life?** Changing your lifestyle takes time and effort.

Do you need help with personal responsibilities, so you can free up time to work out, attend a group meeting or cook a healthy meal?

Who can help you around the house or at work so that you will have more time to make the changes you need?

## KEYS TO A SUCCESSFUL PARTNERSHIP

🍎 First you must set realistic goals. Let family and friends know how important making a particular change is to you. Let them know you are committed to success.

🍎 When asking for help, be as specific as you can—tell others exactly how they can help you. Better yet, work out a plan together and develop a contract.

🍎 Communicate openly and often about your thoughts, feelings and needs. Practice positive communication—avoid being negative or critical.

🍎 Never expect one person to be *all things* for you.

🍎 Be sensitive to the needs of others. Always consider how you can help those who help you. Don't hesitate to ask for the help you need, but try to offer something in return. Reward others for their help—say thank-you, buy them small gifts or treat them to special occasions.

---

## A CONTRACT FOR PARTNERSHIP

My goal—what I need you to help me accomplish:


Steps I will take to help me reach my goal:


My reward for reaching my goal:


This is what I need you to do to help me reach my goal:


Steps you will take to help me reach my goal:


Your reward for helping me reach my goal:


_____          _____
           Signature                        Date

---

# PREVENTING
# HEART DISEASE

Diseases of the heart and blood vessels—cardiovascular disease—claim nearly 1 million lives in the United States each year. That's one death every three seconds! Coronary heart disease (CHD), which causes heart attacks, is the leading killer of both men and women. Each year over 1 million heart attacks occur and nearly 500,000 result in death—one-half of these victims are women! Stroke, another form of cardiovascular disease, is the third leading killer of men and women.

## THE CAUSES OF HEART ATTACKS AND STROKES

Arteriosclerosis is the underlying process that causes most heart disease. It results from the buildup of fat, cholesterol and cells in the lining of the arteries. This buildup is called plaque and as it progresses, the flow of blood to the heart or brain can be blocked, or the plaque can rupture, causing a heart attack or stroke. While heart attack and stroke can occur suddenly, the process actually develops over many years.

### The Eight Major Risk Factors

There are now eight major risk factors for heart disease. The more factors a person has, the greater the risk of heart attack and stroke. Notice that the first two are factors that cannot be changed, but the rest are changes you can make in your lifestyle.

1. **Age**—Men aged 45 or older and women 55 and older are at a higher risk. The risk for women seems to increase most dramatically after menopause.

   What is your age? _____

2. **Family History**—Your risk is higher if you have a family history of coronary heart disease—a male relative who had a heart attack before the age of 55 or female relative before the age of 65.

Do you have a family history of coronary disease? ☐ Yes ☐ No

3. **Smoking**—A smoker's risk of heart attack is twice that of a non-smoker. Secondhand smoke also increases your risk. A smoker is much more likely to die when a heart attack or stroke occurs than a nonsmoker. If you smoke, make every possible effort to quit.

   Are you currently a smoker? ☐ Yes ☐ No

4. **Abnormal Cholesterol Levels**—The risk of heart disease rises as the total and LDL cholesterol (the *bad* cholesterol) levels increase. The risk of heart disease also rises as HDL cholesterol (the *good* cholesterol) levels decrease. High triglycerides may also increase your risk.

   What are your cholesterol levels? Write them in the appropriate boxes.

| Risk | Low | | Borderline | | High | |
|------|-----|--|------------|--|------|--|
| | Range | My Score | Range | My Score | Range | My Score |
| Total Cholesterol | <200 | | 200-239 | | ≥ 240 | |
| LDL Cholesterol | <130 | | 130-159 | | ≥ 160 | |
| HDL Cholesterol | >35 | | | | ≤ 35 | |
| Triglycerides | <200 | | | | ≥ 200 | |

   If your numbers are in the high or borderline range and you have two or more other risk factors, you may be greatly adding to your risk of a heart attack or stroke. Talk to your doctor. Treatment and prevention always involve lifestyle changes such as following a diet low in saturated fat and cholesterol, achieving and maintaining a desirable weight, and regular physical activity.

5. **High Blood Pressure**—High blood pressure increases the risk of heart attack and stroke. A blood pressure greater than 140/90 is high. Even pressures slightly lower—135-139/85-89—can put you at greater risk.

   **What's your blood pressure?** Write your blood pressure in the appropriate box.

| Risk | Low | Borderline | High |
|------|-----|------------|------|
| Scale | <135/85 | | ≥ 140/90 |
| My Blood Pressure | | | |

If your blood pressure is high, talk to your doctor. Treatment and prevention always involve lifestyle changes such as weight control, physical activity and restriction of alcohol and sodium intake. An eating plan high in fruits and vegetables (7 to 10 servings a day) and low-fat dairy products (2 to 3 servings a day) may also help lower blood pressure.

6. **Physical Inactivity**—A sedentary lifestyle increases the risk of heart disease nearly two times. This risk is as high as that caused by abnormal cholesterol levels, high blood pressure and cigarette smoking combined. Despite the known risks, 60 percent of adults and 30 percent of children don't get enough physical activity to benefit their health. Regular moderate physical activity cuts your risk of dying from heart disease in half.

   Are you getting at least 30 minutes of moderate physical activity several days each week? ☐ Yes ☐ No

7. **Obesity and Overweight**—Excess body fat increases the risk for both heart attack and stroke. Obesity is also associated with increased blood pressure, abnormal cholesterol levels and diabetes. Losing just 10 percent of excess weight and keeping it off can significantly lower risk.

   Are you within your healthy weight range? ☐ Yes ☐ No

8. **Diabetes**—Diabetes (high blood sugar) is very damaging to the heart and blood vessels. If you or a loved one has diabetes, it's important to do all you can to control blood sugar and other risk factors. A fasting blood sugar level greater than 125 mg/dL puts you at risk for heart disease. Many First Place members have been able to reduce the amount of diabetes medications after adopting a healthy lifestyle.

   What's your fasting blood sugar level? _____

# UNDERSTANDING VITAMINS AND MINERALS

When it comes to vitamins and minerals, does it seem that information is changing faster than you can keep up with it? If you're like most people, you probably have many questions: Do I need to take supplements for good health? If so, which ones do I need? How much do I need? How much is too much? Do supplements contain what they say they do? Who and what should I believe?

It's true—recommendations are changing. The National Academy of Sciences is updating its recommendations on vitamins and minerals. You may hear about Dietary Reference Intakes (DRIs), Recommended Dietary Allowances (RDAs) and the Tolerable Upper Intake Level (**UL**). Now experts are looking at what levels of vitamins and minerals are necessary to both prevent disease and promote good health, and how much is too much. RDAs are the dietary intakes that meet the nutritional requirements of nearly all individuals, and the UL is the maximum safe level of daily intake.

The following tables will help you get a better understanding of vitamins and minerals—what they do, how much is recommended (DRIs or RDAs), common doses in supplements, Tolerable Upper Intake Level (UL) when available and, most importantly, the best food sources (nothing replaces God's good food). When it comes to vitamins and mineral supplements, you have to decide what's right for you.

**First Place advises that you discuss the issue of vitamin and mineral supplementation with your personal physician.**

# VITAMINS

There are 13 vitamins—four fat-soluble (A,D,E and K) and nine water soluble (C and the B vitamins). Compared to the major nutrients—carbohydrates, fats, proteins, and water—vitamins are only needed in small amounts, and they are not a source of energy for the body.

| | ROLES AND FACTS | COMMON DOSAGES | GOOD SOURCES |
|---|---|---|---|
| Vitamin A | Maintains healthy cells, skin, and bones; important for vision and immune function. High doses can damage the liver. It's easy to get all the vitamin A you need from a healthy diet. | Women: 800 mcg[1] RE[2] (4,000 IU[3]). Men: 1,000 mcg RE (5,000 IU)—Avoid supplements exceeding the RDA. | Dairy products (cheese, butter, egg yolks); liver; fish oil; fortified foods; and dark green, yellow and orange vegetables. |
| Beta-carotene (Carotenoids) | Beta-carotene from plant sources is converted to vitamin A. Beta-carotene is an antioxidant that may protect the body from heart disease, cancer and cataracts. | No RDA—Supplements range from 2,500 to 25,000 IU (1.5-15 mg[4]). | Look for fruits and vegetables with orange, red, yellow or dark green color (carrots, sweet potatoes, spinach, red bell pepper, apricots, mangoes and cantaloupe). |

| | Roles and Facts | Common Dosages | Good Sources |
|---|---|---|---|
| Vitamin C | Antioxidant that protects your body's cells. Important for healthy skin, connective tissue, bone, and immune function. Large doses increase the risk of kidney stones. | 60 mg—Supplements range from 60 to 500 mg. | All citrus fruits, cantaloupe, strawberries, tomatoes, red and green bell peppers, potatoes and broccoli. It's easy to get what you need. |
| Vitamin D | Helps your body absorb calcium and phosphorous and build healthy bones. Too much vitamin D can cause kidney damage and weaken bones. | 5 to 15 mcg (200-600 IU)—Supplements range from 100 to 800 IU. **UL is 50 mcg (2,000 IU)**. | Vitamin D is formed by the action of sunlight on the skin. Most milk products are fortified. Eggs, fish, margarine and fortified cereals also contain vitamin D. |
| Vitamin E | An antioxidant that protects your body's cells. It may protect against heart disease and cancer. It's been *claimed* to cure almost anything and slow the aging process. | Women: 8mg (12 IU); Men: 10 mg (15 IU)—Supplements range from RDA to 400 IU. | Vegetable oils, nuts, seeds, salad dressings, margarine, wheat germ and green leafy vegetables. |

| | Roles and Facts | Common Dosages | Good Sources |
|---|---|---|---|
| Vitamin K | Important for blood clotting; a deficiency of vitamin K is very unlikely because your body produces it from bacteria in the intestines and it's abundant in food. | Women: 65 mcg; Men: 80 mcg—No need to supplement. | Green leafy vegetables such as spinach and broccoli, peas, eggs, meat, milk, cereal and fruits. |
| Thiamin (Vitamin B1) | All B vitamins are important for energy production, metabolism and building healthy cells (proteins, blood and nerves). | Women: 1.1 mg; Men: 1.2 mg—Appears to be nontoxic. | Whole grains, fortified cereals, enriched grains, nuts, seeds and meats. |
| Riboflavin (Vitamin B2) | Same as thiamin. | Women: 1.1 mg; Men: 1.3 mg—Appears to be nontoxic. | Whole grains, fortified cereals, enriched grains, nuts, seeds, meats, dairy products and green leafy vegetables. |
| Niacin | High doses used *under doctor supervision* to treat high cholesterol levels. | Women: 14 mg; Men: 16 mg—UL is 35 mg. | Same as riboflavin, but meats are the best source. |

| | Roles and Facts | Common Dosages | Good Sources |
|---|---|---|---|
| Vitamin B6 (Pyridoxine) | May reduce levels of homocysteine, which is associated with heart attack and stroke. High doses can cause nerve damage. | Women: 1.3-1.5 mg; Men: 1.3-1.7 mg—Supplements range from RDA to 50 mg. **UL is 100 mg.** | Same as riboflavin. |
| Folate | Very important in pregnancy; may reduce levels of homocysteine which is associated with heart attack and stroke. | 400 mcg—**UL for supplementation is 1,000 mcg.** | Same as riboflavin; legumes and fortified cereals are important sources. |
| Vitamin B12 | May reduce levels of homocysteine which is associated with heart attack and stroke. | 2.4 mcg—Appears to be nontoxic. | Animal and fortified foods only. |
| Biotin | | 30 mcg—Supplements range from 30 to 100 mcg. | Found in a wide variety of foods. |
| Pantothenic Acid | | 30 mcg—Appears to be nontoxic. | Found in a wide variety of foods. |

Notes   1. mcg = micrograms   2. RE = retinol equivalence   3. IU = international units   4. mg = milligrams

# MINERALS

There are probably over 60 minerals in the body. Just like vitamins, minerals play many important roles in the body.

| | ROLES AND FACTS | COMMON DOSAGES | GOOD SOURCES |
|---|---|---|---|
| Calcium | Necessary for healthy bones. Plays an important role in muscle and nerve function and blood clotting. Low calcium intake increases the risk for osteoporosis. High calcium intake can cause kidney stones. | 800-1200 mg—Aim for 1,200 mg. Supplements range from 250 to 1500 mg. UL is 2,500 mg. | Milk and dairy products (yogurt and cheese); dark green leafy vegetables; fortified foods such as juice, some cereals—tofu and soy milk are also good sources. |
| Chloride | Helps regulate fluid balance; important in digestion and nerve function. | No RDA—No need to supplement. | Salt. |
| Chromium | Works with insulin to regulate blood sugar. Studies don't support its role in promoting weight loss. | No RDA—Supplements range from 50 to 200 mcg. | Meat, eggs, whole grains and cheese. |

| | ROLES AND FACTS | COMMON DOSAGES | GOOD SOURCES |
|---|---|---|---|
| Copper | Important in red blood cell formation and is a part of many enzymes. | No RDA—Supplements range from 1 to 3 mg. | Seafood, nuts and seeds. |
| Flouride | Important for healthy bones and teeth. | Women: 3.1 mg; Men: 3.8 mg—Supplements range from 1.5 to 4 mg. **UL is 10 mg.** | Fluoridated drinking water and seafood. |
| Iodine | An important part of thyroid hormone which regulates metabolism. | 150 mcg—Intakes of up to 2-3 mg appear safe. | Salt, seafood and some vegetables. |
| Iron | Needed to carry oxygen in the blood; avoid taking supplements with high doses of iron, unless prescribed by doctor. | Women:10 to 15 mg; Men:10 mg. | Meats (the redder and darker the meat, the higher the iron), fortified cereals and grains, beans, nuts, seeds and dried fruits. |
| Magnesium | Important for healthy bones, nerves and muscles; a component of many enzymes. | Women: 320 mg; Men: 420 mg—**UL for supplementation is 350 mg.** | Legumes, nuts, whole grains and leafy green vegetables. |

| | Roles and Facts | Common Dosages | Good Sources |
|---|---|---|---|
| Manganese | Component of many enzymes. | No RDA—supplements range from 2 to 5 mg. | Whole grains, fruits and vegetables and tea. |
| Molybdenum | Component of many enzymes. | No RDA—supplements range from 75 to 250 mcg. | Milk, legumes and whole grains. |
| Phospherous | Important for healthy bones and teeth—helps regulate energy and maintain healthy cells. | 700 mg: UL is 3,000 to 4,000 mg. | Dairy products, meats, legumes, nuts and eggs. |
| Potassium | Helps regulate fluid balance; important in muscle and nerve function. | No RDA—Supplements may contain 2,000 mg. | Fruits, vegetables and meats. |
| Selenium | Antioxidant that protects body's cells. May be protective against some cancers. | Women: 55 mcg; Men: 70 mcg. | Seafood, meats and eggs; grains, nuts and seeds may also contain selenium. |
| Sodium | Helps regulate fluid balance; important in muscle and nerve function. A diet high in sodium may promote high blood pressure. | No RDA—No need to supplement. Limit to 2,400 mg/day. | Salt and processed foods. |

| | Roles and Facts | Common Dosages | Good Sources |
|---|---|---|---|
| Zinc | Important for cell growth, immune function, wound healing and energy metabolism. | Women: 12 mg; Men: 15 mg. | Meat, seafood, whole grains, nuts, seeds, milk and eggs. |

## Summary and Notes

It's important to try to meet your body's need for vitamins and minerals by following a healthy eating plan. If you decide that taking a supplement is right for you, it's best to stick with a multivitamin and mineral supplement that provides no more than the DRIs or RDAs. There is no evidence that taking higher doses of certain vitamins and minerals is necessary for good health. Whatever you do, try not to take supplements with vitamins and minerals in excess of the highest dosages listed in the tables above.

It's important to note that the above common dosages are for healthy adults only; these levels may not be appropriate for children and adolescents.

If you're pregnant, breast-feeding your child or thinking about becoming pregnant, discuss your nutritional needs with your personal physician. The common dosages listed may not be appropriate if you're pregnant or breast-feeding your child.

The above common dosages may not apply to elderly individuals or people with underlying health problems. If you think you may have special nutritional needs, talk with your personal physician before taking any vitamin or mineral supplements.

Many vitamin and mineral supplements list the % Daily Value on the Nutrition Facts Panel. Use the tables above when you're unsure about the amount of a particular vitamin or mineral in a supplement.

# WINNING OVER WORRY

*Who of you by worrying can add a single hour to his life?* Matthew 6:27

Do worry and stress ever interfere with the quality of your life? Do they sometimes make it difficult for you to experience the *abundant* life that Christ desires for you? Are daily responsibilities such as work, home life, finances and service, wearing you down? If you can answer yes to any of these questions, chances are worry is taking a toll on your health, happiness and effectiveness. But it doesn't have to be that way—God has a plan for you:

Cast all your anxiety on him because he cares for you (1 Peter 5:7).

God's Word repeatedly tells us not to worry or be anxious. Read the following verses, putting your name in the blanks:

_____, do not be anxious about anything, but in everything, by prayer and petition, with thanksgiving, present your requests to God. And the peace of God, which transcends all understanding, will guard your heart and mind in Christ Jesus (see Philippians 4:6,7).

_____, peace I leave with you; my peace I give you. I do not give to you as the world gives. _____, do not let your heart be troubled and do not be afraid (see John 14:27).

Meditate on these verses. Breathe deeply as you think about "peace," "do not be anxious" and "do not let your [heart] be troubled." Try to fill your lungs from the top to the bottom, and as you breathe out, feel your muscles relax. Chances are you're feeling better already: physically, mentally, emotionally and spiritually. What you're experiencing is the relaxation response—God's design for helping the body overcome the effects of worry, stress and anxiety.

## WORRY: COUNTING THE COST

The stress and strain of worry

- Draws your focus away from God;
- Can interfere with important relationships;
- Affects you mentally, emotionally, spiritually and physically;
- Leaves you feeling fatigued;
- Suppresses the immune system;
- Causes headaches, digestive problems, sleeplessness and depression;
- Might also encourage unhealthy habits such as a poor diet and physical inactivity.

## IDENTIFY THE WORRIES AND STRESSES IN YOUR LIFE

Many things in life cause worry, stress and anxiety. Many times our worries are very real: pressures at work, too much responsibility at home and financial difficulties. Other times worry only exists in the mind and imagination. However, too often we worry about things that will never come to pass.

What things cause you to feel stressed or worried? Are you doing all you can to eliminate or respond positively to the worries in your life? Are you trusting God to deliver you from your worries? God never promises that you will not experience difficult times, but He does offer a way out:

Come to me, all you who are weary and burdened, and I will give you rest. Take my yoke upon you and learn from me, for I am gentle and humble in heart, and you will find rest for your souls. For my yoke is easy and my burden is light (Matthew 11:28-30).

# A Plan for Winning over Worry and Stress

God's prescription for overcoming worry is found in Philippians 4:6-9: prayer and thankfulness (v. 7), right thinking (v. 8) and action (v. 9). Here are some things you can do to take control of the worry and stress in your life.

## Take Life One Day at a Time

> Therefore do not worry about tomorrow, for tomorrow will worry about itself. Each day has enough trouble of its own (Matthew 6:34).

Are you managing your time well? Are your goals in line with God's purpose for your life? Are you making time in your life for the important things? Jesus doesn't tell us not to *think* about tomorrow; He tells us not to *worry* about tomorrow! Planning and preparing will help eliminate stress and worry. Keeping a calendar or schedule can help you control stress and organize your time. Learn to say no more often and eliminate those things that are less important. Keep the big picture of your life in front of you and don't get discouraged by the small setbacks that happen along the way.

## Take Time to Rest and Relax

> Come with me by yourselves to a quiet place and get some rest (Mark 6:31).

Are you taking time each day for rest and relaxation? Take at least 15 to 20 minutes every day to do something relaxing: sit quietly, breathe deeply, take a walk, read, meditate and/or pray. The relaxation exercise you did at the beginning of this handout is a great way to get started. Choose meaningful Scripture verses that work for you. Progressive relaxation involves tightening and relaxing each muscle group in your body as you lie comfortably and breathe deeply. You can also use mental imagery to relax—imagine a soothing scene in your mind while listening to peaceful music. Choose what works best for you.

## Take Care of Yourself

> Do you not know that your body is a temple of the Holy Spirit, who
> is in you, whom you have received from God? You are not your own;
> you were bought at a price. Therefore honor God with your body
> (1 Corinthians 6:19,20).

Are you making time for regular physical activity, following a healthy eating plan and getting adequate sleep? Do your poor health habits or feelings about your body contribute to the worry in your life? Physical activity is a great way to relieve stress and worry. A physically fit body responds better to the stresses of life. Regular endurance exercise may even trigger the relaxation response by releasing feel-good hormones called "endorphins." Do what you enjoy: walk, swim, ride a bike or jog. Any activity that gets your muscles moving and increases your heart rate can be helpful.

## Build Supportive Relationships

> A friend loves at all times and a brother is born for adversity
> (Proverbs 17:27).

Do you have a close network of family and friends who can help you in time of stress? Sharing your worries can make you feel better and help you put things in perspective. Make sure you establish supportive relationships with *positive* people to help you in times of stress. Share your burdens and concerns with others and ask for help when you need it.

# TWO WEEKS OF MENU PLANS

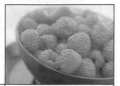

## FIRST PLACE MENU PLANS

*Each plan is based on approximately 1400 calories.*

| | |
|---|---|
| Breakfast | 2 breads, 1 fruit, 1 milk, 0-½ fat |
| | (When a meat exchange is used, milk is omitted.) |
| Lunch | 2 meats, 2 breads, 1 vegetable, 1 fruit, 1 fat |
| Dinner | 3 meats, 2 breads, 2 vegetables, 1 fat |
| Snacks | 1 bread, 1 fruit, 1 milk, ½-1 fat (or any remaining exchanges) |

*For more calories, add the following to the 1400 calorie plan.*

| | |
|---|---|
| 1600 calories | Add 2 breads, 1 fat |
| 1800 calories | 2 meats, 3 breads, 1 vegetable, 1 fat |
| 2000 calories | 2 meats, 4 breads, 1 vegetable, 3 fats |
| 2200 calories | 2 meats, 5 breads, 1 vegetable, 1 fruit, 5 fats |
| 2400 calories | 2 meats, 6 breads, 2 vegetables, 1 fruit, 6 fats |

The exchanges for these meals were calculated using the MasterCook software. It uses a database of over 6,000 food items prepared using United States Department of Agriculture (USDA) publications and information from food manufacturers. As with any nutritional program, MasterCook calculates the nutritional values of the recipes based on ingredients. Nutrition may vary due to how the food is prepared, where the food comes from, i.e., geography, soil content, season, ripeness, processing and method of preparation. For these reasons, please use the recipes and menu plans as approximate guides. As always consult your physician and/or a registered dietician before starting a diet program.

## 🍎 Breakfasts

2 Eggo low-fat waffles
½ cup unsweetened applesauce (to top waffle)
1 pack Sweet & Low (to sweeten applesauce)
2 tbsp. raisins
1 cup nonfat milk
**Exchanges: 2 breads, 2 fruits, 1 milk**

~~~~~~~~~~~~~~~~~~~~~~~~~~~~~~~~~~~~~~~~~~~~~~~~~~~~~~~

1 package instant flavored oatmeal with 4 walnut halves, chopped
½ banana
1 cup nonfat milk
**Exchanges: 2 breads, 1 fruit, 1 milk, ½ fat**

~~~~~~~~~~~~~~~~~~~~~~~~~~~~~~~~~~~~~~~~~~~~~~~~~~~~~~~

1 medium reduced-fat oat muffin
1 medium fresh peach or other fruit
1 cup nonfat artificially sweetened fruit-flavored yogurt
**Exchanges: 2 breads 1 fruit 1 milk ½ fat**

~~~~~~~~~~~~~~~~~~~~~~~~~~~~~~~~~~~~~~~~~~~~~~~~~~~~~~~

¾ cup Rice Chex cereal
1 cup nonfat milk
½ banana
½ English muffin
½ tsp. margarine
1 tsp. all-fruit spread
**Exchanges: 2 breads, 1 fruit, 1 milk, ½ fat**

~~~~~~~~~~~~~~~~~~~~~~~~~~~~~~~~~~~~~~~~~~~~~~~~~~~~~~~

⅓ medium cantaloupe or honeydew melon
1 cup nonfat artificially sweetened pineapple-flavored yogurt (to top melon)
¼ cup Grape-Nuts cereal (sprinkled on yogurt)
**Exchanges: 1½ breads, 1 fruit, 1 milk**

~~~~~~~~~~~~~~~~~~~~~~~~~~~~~~~~~~~~~~~~~~~~~~~~~~~~~~~

1 cup fortified cold cereal
½ small mango
1 cup nonfat milk
**Exchanges: 2 breads, 1 fruit, 1 milk**

~~~~~~~~~~~~~~~~~~~~~~~~~~~~~~~~~~~~~~~~~~~~~~~~~~

1 small (2-oz.) bagel
1 tsp. strawberry jam
1 cup aspartame-sweetened, mixed-berry nonfat yogurt
¾ cup blackberries (mix into yogurt)
**Exchanges: 2 breads, 1 fruit, 1 milk**

~~~~~~~~~~~~~~~~~~~~~~~~~~~~~~~~~~~~~~~~~~~~~~~~~~

1 cup puffed rice cereal
½ medium banana, sliced
1 cup nonfat milk
**Exchanges: 2 breads, 1 fruit, 1 milk**

~~~~~~~~~~~~~~~~~~~~~~~~~~~~~~~~~~~~~~~~~~~~~~~~~~

1 small (2-oz.) English muffin
1 tsp. reduced-calorie margarine
½ medium grapefruit
1 cup nonfat milk
**Exchanges: 2 breads, 1 fruit, 1 milk, ½ fat**

~~~~~~~~~~~~~~~~~~~~~~~~~~~~~~~~~~~~~~~~~~~~~~~~~~

1 cup wheat flakes cereal
1 medium peach, sliced
1 cup nonfat milk
**Exchanges: 2 breads, 1 fruit, 1 milk**

~~~~~~~~~~~~~~~~~~~~~~~~~~~~~~~~~~~~~~~~~~~~~~~~~~

1 small (2 oz.) bagel, toasted
1 tsp. reduced-calorie tub margarine
¾ cup raspberries
1 cup nonfat milk
**Exchanges: 2 breads, 1 fruit, 1 milk, ½ fat**

~~~~~~~~~~~~~~~~~~~~~~~~~~~~~~~~~~~~~~~~~~~~~~~~~~

1 cup bran flakes cereal
2 tbsp. raisins
1 cup nonfat milk
**Exchanges: 2 breads, 1 fruit, 1 milk**

~~~~~~~~~~~~~~~~~~~~~~~~~~~~~~~~~~~~~~~~~~~~~~~~~~

2 frozen pancakes, heated

2 tsp. diet syrup

½ medium grapefruit

1 cup nonfat milk

**Exchanges: 2 breads, 1 fruit, 1 milk, ½ fat**

~~~~~~~~~~~~~~~~~~~~~~~~~~~~~~~~~~~~~~~~~~~~~~~~~~~

2 slices reduced-calorie wheat bread, toasted

2 tsp. reduced-calorie tub margarine

¾ oz. raisin bran cereal

1 cup strawberries

½ cup nonfat milk

**Exchanges: 2 breads, 1 fruit, 1 milk, ½ fat**

~~~~~~~~~~~~~~~~~~~~~~~~~~~~~~~~~~~~~~~~~~~~~~~~~~~

## 🍎 LUNCHES

### Turkey Salad

Combine 2 oz. skinless boneless cooked turkey breast, diced, ¼ cup chopped celery, 2 tbsp. each chopped red onion and spinach leaves, 1 tsp. fresh lemon juice and 2 tsp. reduced-calorie mayonnaise.

**Serve with** ½ cup each tomato and cucumber slices, 2 tsp. lite Italian dressing, 2 rice cakes and 1 pear.

**Exchanges: 2 meats, 2 breads, 1 vegetable, 1 fruit, 1 fat**

~~~~~~~~~~~~~~~~~~~~~~~~~~~~~~~~~~~~~~~~~~~~~~~~~~~

### Broiled Flounder

3 oz. flounder, broiled

**Serve with** ¾ cup boiled new potatoes with 1 tsp. reduced-calorie margarine and minced fresh parsley, 1 cup steamed zucchini slices, 1 iceberg lettuce wedge, 1 tbsp. reduced-fat Thousand Island dressing, a 1-oz. breadstick and a small orange.

**Exchanges: 2 meats, 2 breads, 1 vegetable, 1 fruit, 1 fat**

~~~~~~~~~~~~~~~~~~~~~~~~~~~~~~~~~~~~~~~~~~~~~~~~~~~

## Broccoli Bisque

In food processor, combine 2 cups frozen chopped broccoli and $\frac{1}{2}$ cup low-sodium chicken broth and $\frac{1}{2}$ cup nonfat milk; puree until smooth. Transfer to medium saucepan; cook until heated. Season with salt and pepper if desired.

Serve with 1 small apple and **Egg Salad Muffin**. In small bowl, combine 2 hard-cooked egg whites, chopped; 1 hard-cooked egg, chopped; 1 tbsp. finely chopped celery and 2 tsp. reduced-calorie mayonnaise; scoop onto a toasted English muffin.

**Exchanges:** 2 meats, 2 breads, 2 vegetables, 1 fruit, 1 fat

~~~~~~~~~~~~~~~~~~~~~~~~~~~~~~~~~~~~~~~~~~~~~~~~~~~~~~

## Tuna Salad Nicoise

In medium bowl, combine 2 cups shredded romaine lettuce leaves, 1 medium tomato, quartered, $\frac{1}{2}$ cup cooked cut green beans, 4 oz. drained canned water-packed tuna, drained; 4 large pitted black olives and 1 tbsp. reduced-fat Italian dressing.

Serve with 2 long breadsticks and 1 banana.

**Exchanges:** 2 meats, 2 breads, 2 vegetables, 1 fruit, 1 fat

~~~~~~~~~~~~~~~~~~~~~~~~~~~~~~~~~~~~~~~~~~~~~~~~~~~~~~

## Bean and Salsa Salad

In small bowl, combine $\frac{1}{2}$ cup drained cooked red kidney beans, $1\frac{1}{2}$ oz. shredded pepper jack cheese, $\frac{1}{2}$ cup finely chopped red onion, $\frac{1}{4}$ cup salsa and 1 tsp. fresh lime juice. Line plate with spinach leaves; top with bean mixture, 2 tbsp. reduced fat sour cream and 1 tsp. minced fresh cilantro.

Serve with 1 oz. nonfat tortilla chips and $\frac{1}{2}$ small mango.

**Exchanges:** 2 meats, 2 breads, 1 vegetable, 1 fruit, 1 fat

~~~~~~~~~~~~~~~~~~~~~~~~~~~~~~~~~~~~~~~~~~~~~~~~~~~~~~

## Cottage Cheese Lunch

One-half cup 2% cottage cheese topped with $\frac{1}{4}$ cup each chopped tomato and alfalfa sprouts and $\frac{1}{2}$ tbsp. chopped scallions.

Serve with $\frac{1}{2}$ cup each red and green bell pepper strips with 2 tbsp. reduced-fat ranch dressing; 2 slices reduced-calorie rye bread, toasted;

2 tsp. reduced-calorie tub margarine; 2 plums and 4 oz. sugar-free chocolate nonfat frozen yogurt.
**Exchanges: 2 meats, 2 breads, 1 vegetable, 1 fruit, 1 fat**

~~~~~~~~~~~~~~~~~~~~~~~~~~~~~~~~~~~~~~~~~~~~~~~~~~~~~~

## Tuna-Pasta Salad

In medium bowl, combine ½ cup cooked shell macaroni, 4 oz. drained canned water-packed white tuna, 6 cherry tomatoes, halved, ¼ cup diced red onion and 1 tbsp. reduced-fat Italian dressing.

**Serve with** ½ cup each carrot and celery sticks, 1 oz. whole-wheat roll with 1 tsp. reduced-calorie margarine and 1 medium peach.
**Exchanges: 2 meats, 2 breads, 1 vegetable, 1 fruit, 1 fat**

~~~~~~~~~~~~~~~~~~~~~~~~~~~~~~~~~~~~~~~~~~~~~~~~~~~~~~

## Spinach-Mushroom Salad

In medium bowl, combine 2 cups torn spinach leaves, ¼ cup each sliced mushrooms and sliced red onion, 1 hard-cooked egg, sliced, 2 tsp. imitation bacon bits and 2 tbsp. lite Italian dressing.

**Serve with** ½ cup each celery and carrot sticks, 1 small peach and 2 long breadsticks.
**Exchanges: 1 meat, 2 breads, 2 vegetables, 1 fruit, 1 fat**

~~~~~~~~~~~~~~~~~~~~~~~~~~~~~~~~~~~~~~~~~~~~~~~~~~~~~~

## Broiled Ham and Cheese Sandwich

Toast 2 slices reduced-calorie whole-wheat bread; layer ½ oz. thinly sliced cooked ham, 2 tomato slices and ½ slice nonfat, processed American cheese onto each toast slice. Place onto nonstick baking sheet; broil until cheese melts.

**Serve with** 1 small pear and **Bean Salad**. In small bowl, combine ⅓ cup each steamed green beans, sugar snap peas and wax beans, and 1 tbsp. reduced-fat Italian dressing.
**Exchanges: 2 meats, 1 bread, 2 vegetables, 1 fruit, 1 fat**

~~~~~~~~~~~~~~~~~~~~~~~~~~~~~~~~~~~~~~~~~~~~~~~~~~~~~~

## Shrimp Salad

In small bowl, combine 2½ oz. peeled and deveined cooked shrimp, chopped; 2 tsp. reduced-calorie mayonnaise, ½ tsp. chili sauce, ½ tsp. each fresh lemon juice and sweet pickle relish.

**Serve with** ½ cup each carrot and celery sticks, 2 cups watercress or romaine leaves with 6 cherry tomatoes, 1 cup sliced cucumber and 2 tbsp. reduced fat Italian dressing, 1 2-oz. toasted bagel with 1 tsp. reduced-calorie margarine and 15 grapes.

**Exchanges: 2 meats, 2 breads, 2 vegetables, 1 fruit, 1 fat**

~~~~~~~~~~~~~~~~~~~~~~~~~~~~~~~~~~~~~~~~~~~~~~~~~~~~~~

## Grilled Chicken Salad

In medium bowl, combine 1 cup torn spinach leaves, ½ medium tomato, sliced, ½ medium roasted red bell pepper, sliced, ½ cup mandarin oranges, 2 oz. skinless boneless grilled chicken breast, sliced, 2 tsp. red wine vinegar, 1 tsp. olive oil and freshly ground black pepper, to taste.

**Serve with** 3 melba toast and ½ cup reduced-calorie chocolate-flavored pudding.

**Exchanges: 2 meats, 2 breads, 1 vegetable, 1 fruit, 1 fat**

~~~~~~~~~~~~~~~~~~~~~~~~~~~~~~~~~~~~~~~~~~~~~~~~~~~~~~

## Chicken Noodle Soup

1 cup canned chicken noodle soup
1 cup broccoli florets with 2 tbsp. fat-free ranch dressing
1 slice Velveeta light cheese
8 low-fat saltines
2-inch wedge honeydew melon

**Exchanges: 1 meat, 2 breads, 1 vegetable, 1 fruit, 1 fat**

~~~~~~~~~~~~~~~~~~~~~~~~~~~~~~~~~~~~~~~~~~~~~~~~~~~~~~

## Roast Chicken Breast

2 oz. skinless roast chicken breast, cut into strips
½ cup cooked brown rice with 1 tsp. reduced-calorie margarine
½ cup each steamed whole green beans and julienne carrots with ½ tsp.
   fresh lemon juice
2 cups mixed field green salad with 1 tbsp. fat-free blue cheese dressing
1 slice diet French bread, toasted
1 tsp. reduced-calorie margarine
1 small apple

**Exchanges: 2 meats, 2 breads, 1 vegetable, 1 fruit, 1 fat**

~~~~~~~~~~~~~~~~~~~~~~~~~~~~~~~~~~~~~~~~~~~~~~~~~~~~~~

## Arby's Junior Roast Beef Sandwich

1 cup cole slaw
1 cup mixed melon balls
**Exchanges: 2 meats, 2 breads, 1 vegetable, 1 fruit, 2 fats**

~~~~~~~~~~~~~~~~~~~~~~~~~~~~~~~~~~~~~~~~~~~~~~~~~~~~~~~~~~~~~

## 🍎 DINNERS

### Steak Tacos

1 lime
1 tbsp. taco seasoning
2 6-oz. $\frac{1}{2}$-inch-thick lean sirloin steaks
$\frac{1}{2}$ cup low-fat Colby Jack cheese, shredded
Lite sour cream

8 6-inch low-fat
   flour tortillas
Shredded lettuce
1 cup prepared salsa

Squeeze lime juice over all surfaces of meat. Sprinkle each side of meat with taco seasoning. Place steaks on a grill over a medium hot fire or under broiler. Grill or broil to desired doneness (4 minutes each side for medium). While steaks are cooking, warm tortillas and salsa. Divide cheese evenly on top of steaks. Cut each steak into 8 pieces. Serve 2 pieces of steak with a tortilla and salsa. Garnish with shredded lettuce and light sour cream. Serves 4.

**Serve with** $\frac{3}{4}$ cup grilled fresh pineapple wedges or canned spears and 1 cup sliced cucumbers marinated in light Italian dressing per person.
**Exchanges: 3 meats, 2$\frac{1}{2}$ breads, 2 vegetables, 1 fruit, 2 fats**

~~~~~~~~~~~~~~~~~~~~~~~~~~~~~~~~~~~~~~~~~~~~~~~~~~~~~~~~~~~~~

### Chicken Breast with Raspberry Sauce

2 tsp. olive oil
1 red onion, thinly sliced
4 4-oz. boneless chicken
   breast with skin
2$\frac{1}{2}$ cups fresh or 1 cup frozen raspberries

$\frac{1}{2}$ tsp. salt
$\frac{1}{4}$ tsp. freshly ground
   black pepper
1 cup raspberry-apple juice

Heat oil in a large nonstick skillet. Add onion; sauté 2 minutes; do not brown. Remove onion and set aside. Season the flesh side of breast with salt and pepper; add to pan and cook over medium heat only until each side is lightly browned. Add juice to pan and continue cooking until chicken is cooked through, about 12 minutes. Remove chicken from pan. Add onions to skillet; cook until liquid has a syrupy consistency. Add raspberries; heat through. Remove skin from chicken before serving and serve breast topped with sauce. Serves 4.

Serve with ⅔ cup cooked rice pilaf and 1 cup steamed broccoli with 1 tsp. melted margarine per person.

Exchanges: 3 meats, 2 breads, 2 vegetables, 1 fruit, 1 fat

~~~~~~~~~~~~~~~~~~~~~~~~~~~~~~~~~~~~~~~~~~~~~~~~~~~~~~

## Mustard Chicken

| | |
|---|---|
| 4 4-oz. boneless chicken breasts | 2 tbsp. Dijon mustard |
| ½ tsp. dried dill | 1 tbsp. olive oil |
| ½ tsp. salt | 2 cloves garlic, minced |
| ¼ tsp. black pepper | ⅓ cup fresh parsley, chopped |
| ½ cup apple cider | ¼ cup water |

Preheat oven to 350° F. On a cutting board cover each breast with plastic wrap and pound with a meat mallet until ½ inch thick. Heat oil in a large nonstick skillet, add garlic and cook for 2 minutes over medium heat. Add chicken breasts and brown 3 minutes on each side. Transfer chicken to a 1½-quart shallow casserole. Put cider, water, mustard, dill, salt and pepper into the skillet; stir to mix with the chicken drippings. Bring to a boil and cook 1 minute. Pour over chicken in casserole. Cover and bake 20 minutes. Add parsley and baste with sauce and bake an additional 5 minutes. Serves 4.

Serve with ½ cup garlic mashed potatoes, 1 cup sautéed squash with peppers and 1 breadstick per person.

Exchanges: 3 meats, 2 breads, 2 vegetables, 1 fat

~~~~~~~~~~~~~~~~~~~~~~~~~~~~~~~~~~~~~~~~~~~~~~~~~~~~~~

## Crock-Pot Cider Pork Stew

| | |
|---|---|
| 2 lbs. lean boneless pork loin | 3 tbsp. flour |
| 1 tsp. salt | ¼ tsp. dried thyme |

¼ tsp. pepper

3 cups carrots, sliced

2 large onions, cubed

2 cups apple cider

½ cup cold water

3 cups potatoes, cubed

2 apples, cubed

1 tbsp. vinegar

¼ cup flour

Cut pork into cubes. Combine the 3 tbsp. of flour, salt, thyme and pepper and toss with meat. Put carrots, potatoes, onion and apple in Crock-Pot. Top with meat cubes. Combine the apple cider and vinegar; pour over meat. Cover and cook on low for 8 to10 hours. Turn Crock-Pot to high. Combine ¼ cup flour and ½ cup cold water and blend well. Stir into liquid in Crock-Pot. Cover and cook 15 to 20 minutes or until thickened. Season to taste. Serves 8.

**Serve with** 2-inch square of cornbread and 1 cup steamed broccoli and cauliflower per person.

**Exchanges: 3 meats, 2 breads, 2 vegetables, 1 fat**

~ ~ ~ ~ ~ ~ ~ ~ ~ ~ ~ ~ ~ ~ ~ ~ ~ ~ ~ ~ ~ ~ ~ ~ ~ ~ ~ ~ ~ ~ ~ ~ ~ ~ ~ ~ ~ ~ ~ ~ ~ ~ ~ ~ ~ ~ ~ ~ ~

## Seared Veal Chops with Sun-Dried Tomatoes

4 lean center-cut veal chops
  (1 ¼ to 1 ½ lbs.)

¼ cup sun-dried tomatoes

1 cup tomato juice

½ cup water

2 tbsp. fresh basil, chopped
  (or 1 tsp. dried leaf basil)

½ tsp. cayenne pepper sauce

salt and pepper to taste

Trim and discard excess fat from chops. In a large frying pan, sear the chops. When the chops are browned on the outside, add the juice, water, hot sauce, salt and pepper. Cover tightly and simmer 15 minutes. Add the sun-dried tomatoes and cook for another 10 minutes. Add ½ of basil and continue to cook for 8 minutes. Add remaining basil and cook for 3 more minutes. To serve, arrange the veal on a plate, and spoon some of the tomatoes and basil over it. Serves 4.

**Serve with** ½ cup Lean Cuisine Pasta Alfredo, ½ cup mixed vegetables and 1 1-oz. dinner roll per person.

**Exchanges: 3 meats, 2 breads, 1 vegetable, 2 fats**

~ ~ ~ ~ ~ ~ ~ ~ ~ ~ ~ ~ ~ ~ ~ ~ ~ ~ ~ ~ ~ ~ ~ ~ ~ ~ ~ ~ ~ ~ ~ ~ ~ ~ ~ ~ ~ ~ ~ ~ ~ ~ ~ ~ ~ ~ ~ ~ ~

# Beef and Noodles in BBQ Sauce

4 oz. fine egg noodles
2 tbsp. reduced-fat margarine
¾ cup onions, diced
1 lb. leanest ground beef
1 lb. mushrooms, sliced

¾ cup water
2 egg yolks
3 tbsp. BBQ sauce
2 tbsp. cooking sherry

Put the noodles into a heat-resistant mixing bowl and cover them with boiling water. Set aside for 20 minutes; then drain. In a frying pan, melt the butter, add the onions and sauté 5 minutes or so. Add the beef, mushrooms and noodles. Increase the heat to high and cook for another 5 minutes, stirring constantly. Add the water and cook another 10 minutes over low heat. In a small bowl, mix together the egg yolks, BBQ sauce and sherry. Scoop a few spoonfuls of the meat mixture into the bowl of egg mixture. Turn the contents of the bowl into the skillet. Heat gently while stirring. Serve over the noodles.

**Serve with** spinach salad topped with croutons and a low-fat dressing.
**Exchanges: 3 meats, 2 breads, 2 vegetables, 2 fats**

# White Turkey Chili

1½ cups onion, chopped
½ cup green bell pepper, chopped
2 cloves garlic, minced
½ tsp. olive oil
1 tsp. cumin
1 17-oz can cannellini beans,
     drained and rinsed
2 cups turkey light meat, cooked and cubed

1 tsp. chili powder
¼ tsp. cayenne pepper
¼ tsp. salt
1 cup chicken broth
1 tsp. oregano

In a 3-quart saucepan over medium heat, cook onions, bell peppers and garlic in oil until tender. Add cumin, oregano, chili powder, cayenne pepper and salt. Cook for 1 minute. Stir in beans and turkey. Bring to a boil; reduce heat and simmer uncovered for 30 minutes or until slightly thickened.

**Serve with** 8 crackers and green salad.
**Exchanges: 3 meats, 2 breads, 1 vegetable, ½ fat**

# Baked Cajun Chicken

1½ to 2 lbs. split chicken breasts
Nonstick spray coating
2 tbsp. nonfat milk
2 tbsp. onion powder

½ tsp. dried thyme, crushed
¼ tsp. garlic salt
⅛ tsp. ground white pepper
⅛ tsp. ground black pepper

Rinse chicken and pat dry. Cut off skin and discard. Spray a 13x9x2-inch baking dish with nonstick cooking spray. Arrange the chicken in the dish, meat side up. Brush lightly with milk. In small bowl mix onion powder, thyme, garlic salt, white pepper, red pepper and black pepper. Sprinkle over chicken. Bake in a 375° F oven for 45 minutes or until the chicken is cooked through.

   **Serve with** ½ cup steamed rice and ½ cup steamed vegetables per person.
**Exchanges: 3 meats, 1 bread, 1 vegetable, 1 fat**

~~~~~~~~~~~~~~~~~~~~~~~~~~~~~~~~~~~~~~~~~~~~~~~~~~~~~~~~~

# Cinnamon Apple Pork Tenderloin

1 lb. pork tenderloin
2 tbsp. cornstarch
2 tbsp. raisins

2 apples, peeled, cored and sliced
1 tsp. ground cinnamon

Preheat the oven to 400° F. Place the pork tenderloin in a roasting pan or casserole dish with a lid. Combine the remaining ingredients in a bowl and stir. Spoon the apple mixture around the pork tenderloin. Cover and bake 40 minutes. Remove the lid and spoon the apple mixture over the tenderloin. Return to the oven and bake 15 to 20 minutes longer until tenderloin is browned and cooked through. Serves 6.

   **Serve with** ½ cup brown rice and 1 cup green beans per person.
**Exchanges: 3 meats, 1 bread, 2 vegetables, 1 fruit**

~~~~~~~~~~~~~~~~~~~~~~~~~~~~~~~~~~~~~~~~~~~~~~~~~~~~~~~~~

# Meat Loaf

1 egg
⅓ cup onion, finely chopped
1 tsp. salt
2 slices bread, finely cubed

2 tbsp. green pepper, finely chopped
1 lb. lean ground round (15% fat or less)
½ tsp. dry mustard
⅓ cup prepared salsa

Preheat oven to 400° F. Mix all ingredients well. Form into a loaf. Place in foil-lined 5x9-inch pan. Bake until done, 40-45 minutes.

**Serve with** ¼ cup mashed potatoes and 1 cup snap peas per person.
**Exchanges: 3 meats, 2 breads, 2 vegetables, 2 fats**

~~~~~~~~~~~~~~~~~~~~~~~~~~~~~~~~~~~~~~~~~~~~~~~~~~~~~~

## Cheese Lasagna

6 oz. whole-wheat lasagna noodles
1 cup onion, bell pepper and
   mushrooms, chopped
   (mix of all three)
1 ½ cups low-fat cottage cheese

1 cup tomato sauce
2 eggs
3 oz. mozzarella cheese, grated
2 tbsp. Parmesan cheese

Cook lasagna noodles in boiling water until tender. Drain and set aside. Combine tomato sauce and chopped onions, peppers and mushrooms. Mix in separate bowl cottage cheese, eggs and half of Parmesan cheese. Preheat oven to 350° F. In a 8x8-inch casserole, layer half the noodles, the cottage cheese mixture and grated mozzarella cheese. Top with tomato sauce mix and the rest of the noodles. Sprinkle with remaining Parmesan cheese. Bake for 25 minutes; then serve hot. Serves 4.
**Exchanges: 3 meats, 2 breads, 1 vegetable, 1 ½ fats**

~~~~~~~~~~~~~~~~~~~~~~~~~~~~~~~~~~~~~~~~~~~~~~~~~~~~~~

## Steamed Shrimp and Scallops

1 lb. shrimp, peeled and deveined
6 oz. sea scallops
¼ cup orange juice
2 tsp. rice vinegar
1 tbsp. oriental sesame oil
½ tsp. dry mustard

½ tsp. salt (or to taste)
¼ tsp. freshly ground black pepper
2 scallions, thinly sliced
1 tbsp. fresh dill, chopped
1 tsp. chives, chopped
4 lettuce leaves

Arrange the shrimp and scallops on a plate in a steamer basket. Sprinkle with 1 tsp. each orange juice and rice vinegar. Place steamer over boiling water in a wok or large skillet and cover. Cook 7 to 8 minutes until shrimp are cooked through. Meanwhile stir together remaining orange juice, rice vinegar, sesame oil, mustard, salt and pepper in a medium bowl. Mix in scallion, dill and chives. Transfer hot seafood to bowl with vinaigrette;

toss to coat well. Serve warm on lettuce-lined plates. Garnish with chopped pimento if desired. Serves 4.

**Serve with** ⅓ steamed corn on the cob, 1 roasted potato and 1 cup green beans per person.

**Exchanges: 3 meats, 2 breads, 2 vegetable, 1 fat**

~~~~~~~~~~~~~~~~~~~~~~~~~~~~~~~~~~~~~~~~~~~~~~~~~~~~~~~~

## Salmon Cakes

1 15½-oz. can red salmon,
  drained (2 cups flaked)
¼ cup red pepper or canned pimiento, diced
6 unsalted-top saltines, crushed

1 tsp. onion powder
4 drops Tabasco sauce
Nonstick cooking spray
3 tbsp. light salad dressing
  or mayonnaise

Remove skin from fish. Combine all ingredients in a medium bowl, mashing salmon bones with a fork. Shape into 4 cakes. Spray a skillet with nonstick cooking spray, and heat over medium heat. Cook salmon cakes, turning once, until lightly browned on each side. Serves 4.

**Serve with** 1 cup cole slaw and 1 breadstick per person.

**Exchanges: 2 ½ meats, 2 breads, 1 vegetable, 1 fat**

~~~~~~~~~~~~~~~~~~~~~~~~~~~~~~~~~~~~~~~~~~~~~~~~~~~~~~~~

## Texas Round Steak

½ cup all-purpose flour
1½ tsp. chili powder
1 lb. 2 oz. round beef, cut into 6 pieces
½ cup fresh green peppers
1 cup fat-free beef broth
1 tsp. chili power

1 tsp. salt
1 tbsp. vegetable oil
½ cup chopped onions
½ cup tomato juice
¼ tsp. garlic powder
⅓ tsp. ground cumin

Blend flour, salt and chili powder well and place in pie pan. Dredge meat in the flour mixture. You should use about half of the mixture. Place oil in a heavy frying pan and heat to frying temperature over moderate heat. Add meat and brown on both sides. Transfer steaks to a 1½-quart casserole. Fry peppers and onions over moderate heat in the pan in which the meat was browned, stirring frequently. Remove vegetables with a slotted spoon and spread over meat. Pour out any remaining fat. Add beef broth to frying pan and cook and stir over moderate heat to loosen brown particles remaining in the pan. Add remaining ingredients to broth. Mix well and pour over meat. Stir the meat and vegetables lightly with a fork to distribute the broth and vegetables. Cover tightly and bake at 325° F for about 1 to 1½ hours or until the meat is tender. Serve some of the sauce with each piece of steak. Serves 6.

**Serve with** 1 cup roasted potatoes and 1 cup sautéed squash per person. **Exchanges: 3 meats, 2 breads, 2 vegetables, 1 fat**

# HEALTHY SNACK CHOICES

| 50-Calorie Snacks | Exchanges |
|---|---|
| 30 small pretzel sticks | 1 bread |
| 1 tangerine | ½ fruit |
| 2 tomatoes | 2 vegetables |
| 1 cup zucchini sticks | 1 vegetable |
| 1 large dill pickle | ½ vegetable |
| 1 4-inch rice cake | ½ bread |
| 1 cup tomato juice | 1½ vegetable |
| 1 carrot | 1½ vegetable |
| 2 gingersnaps | ½ bread, ½ fat |
| ¾ cup raspberries | 1 fruit |
| 12 strawberries | ½ fruit |
| ½ cup fat-free milk | ½ milk |
| 8 celery ribs | 2 vegetable |
| 4 saltine crackers | ½ bread, ½ fat |
| 2 fortune cookies | 1 bread (sugar) |
| 2 cups broccoli flowerets | 2 vegetables |
| 1 kiwi fruit | 1 fruit |
| 3 apricots | 1 fruit |
| ½ cup blueberries | ½ fruit |
| 10 ripe olives | 1 fat |
| ½ cup orange juice | 1 fruit |
| 1 medium cucumber | 2 vegetables |
| 4 slices melba toast | ½ bread |
| 1 medium peach | ½ fruit |
| 1 cup strawberries | ½ fruit |
| 6 cherry tomatoes | 1 vegetable |
| ¾ cup consommé or broth | ½ meat |
| 12 whole radishes | ½ vegetable |
| 1 caramel popcorn cake | 1 bread |
| 2 slices garlic crisp bread | ½ bread |
| ½ cup mandarin orange slices | ½ fruit |
| ¼ cup tropical fruit salad | ½ fruit |

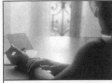

# LEADER DISCUSSION GUIDE

## Week One: Getting Started Right

1.  Begin the session by asking members to share which box they checked on Day 1. Invite group members to share a little about themselves so that others can more fully understand the significance of the box they checked.

2.  Ask a volunteer to read Romans 12:1. Discuss the phrase "offer your bodies as living sacrifices." Ask members to share some practical ways we obey this command. Discuss how we can know we have really done what God says we should do. Does this verse apply only to our attitudes or to specific actions as well?

3.  Refer to Day 3 and Day 4 studies. On the board, write the phrase "The Benefits of a Group." Invite members to suggest the benefits that can be gained by being involved with a support group such as this First Place group. Have a volunteer write on the board the benefits the group identifies.

4.  Invite volunteers to share which box they checked on Day 4 and what they were thinking and feeling that caused them to choose that box.

5.  Have members form groups of three. Ask the groups to identify the ways their health and fitness problems may become a blessing in disguise. Bring the whole group back together and ask members to share some of the key ideas they discussed. Have someone write a summary of these ideas on the board as they share.

6.  **Before the session**, write Philippians 4:13 on a sheet of poster board. Have the group read the verse in unison. Invite members to share a one-sentence concern or fear they have about their potential for success in the First Place program. Then end the sentence with the words of Philippians 4:13. For example, someone might say "I'm afraid I may fail because I've failed in the past, but I can do all things through Him who gives me strength." Encourage each group member to participate in this activity.

7. Ask volunteers to share what changes they will need to make in their lives (from Day 7). Ask if any of them have a stronghold they need to turn over to God. *Note: Don't ask for specifics, unless they volunteer to share. Just ask for a show of hands.*

8. Close in prayer, thanking God that He will give group members the strength they need to overcome any strongholds and be successful in reaching their goals. Encourage each member to select one commitment to work on this week and pray for success in keeping that commitment.

## Week Two: Keeping Commitments

1. **Before the session**, make a poster with the word "Commitment" written at the top with the definition under it (found in the introductory material, p. 22.) Begin the session by directing the group's attention to the poster.

2. Ask volunteers to share with the group which commitment they chose to keep this week and how they did. Ask about problems encountered and how they overcame obstacles. Ask whether they consider their involvement a commitment that they have made to themselves, to others or to God—or to all three.

3. Have someone read Ecclesiastes 5:4. Stress that making a commitment to God is serious (refer to Day 1). Invite members to share how they think God views their involvement in the First Place program and the commitments they have made.

4. Have members form groups of three. Ask groups to list some of the benefits that result from having a serious commitment to God as a central part of the First Place program. Bring the whole group back together and have them report on the benefits they identified. Have a volunteer write the benefits on the board or paper.

5. Read 2 Peter 1:4. Ask volunteers to discuss how and why God's promises are great and precious to them.

6. Ask volunteers to share some of the benefits they have experienced in doing the Bible studies and Scripture memorization as part of the First Place program.

7. Have someone read Psalm 119:11. Discuss how a regular program of Bible study and Scripture memory helps us hide God's Word in our hearts and how God's Word in our hearts helps us resist sin.

8. Close in conversational prayer. Spend the first part of the prayer time thanking God for His Word and the resources He gives us in our everyday lives. Encourage members to reaffirm their commitment to God to work on their goals through His strength.

# Week Three: The Real Enemy

1. Ask three volunteers to quote 1 Peter 5:8, the memory verse for the week.

2. Distribute paper to everyone. Instruct group members to write 1 Peter 5:8 from memory on a piece of paper. Then give them three minutes to analyze this verse and write as many insights, ideas and principles based on this verse as they can write in three minutes. Ask volunteers to share one idea they have written. If necessary, guide the discussion with the following questions: (a) Who is our spiritual enemy? (b) How should we respond to our spiritual enemy? (c) How should the fact that we have an enemy change the way we live? (d) What insights do we gain by the fact that our enemy is compared to a roaring lion? (e) In what ways can Satan devour us?

3. Read 2 Corinthians 10:4. Brainstorm ways that health problems can become a negative stronghold in our lives.

4. Form groups of three. Instruct the groups to share their answers for Day 2. Encourage them to be open and honest so that those in their group will be able to support and pray for them.

5. Have the small groups discuss how a group of friends or a support group can help people deal with negative problems in their lives.

6. Bring the whole group back together. Ask members to share a few of the ways that a support group of friends can help us deal with problems. Discuss why a support group is especially beneficial if a weight problem or lifestyle problem has become a stronghold.

7. Read James 4:7. On the board or paper write "Submit to God and Resist the Devil." Ask the group to name some specific steps we can take to submit to God and resist the devil in our work in the First Place program.

8. Close in prayer. Ask volunteers to pray that they will submit to God and resist the devil this week by praying Scripture verses. Encourage members to thank God that Satan flees from us when we resist him in God's power.

# Week Four: Our Spiritual Weapons

1. **Before the session**, prepare a poster that lists the five spiritual weapons discussed in the study: (a) the name of Jesus; (b) the blood of Jesus; (c) your testimony for Christ; (d) your commitment to Jesus Christ; (e) the Word of God.

2. Affirm that as part of a First Place group, we recognize that success in overcoming health problems depends on spiritual strength. Our first responsibility is to submit to God. Have someone read James 4:7,8. Beginning with the person on your right, ask each person to read one of the commands found in this passage until all five have been read. Ask the group to pray together, expressing their submission to God in all areas of life—especially their physical or health problems.

3. Explain that the spiritual weapons they studied will help them resist Satan and overcome his negative influence in their lives. Form five study groups with at least two people in each group. Assign one spiritual weapon to each group. Instruct the study groups to review the material they studied during the week and prepare a list of practical recommendations for how their spiritual weapon can be used to deal with any lifestyle or health problem. Challenge the groups to be very practical in their recommendations. Make the following assignments: Group 1—the name of Jesus; Group 2—the blood of Jesus; Group 3—your testimony for Christ; Group 4—your commitment to Jesus Christ; Group 5—the Word of God. Allow 10 minutes for the study groups to prepare their recommendations.

4. With the whole group, have one representative from each small group present their recommendations in two minutes or less. After all five groups have reported, give the whole group time to ask any questions about the material presented or to add any comments.

5. As the group members prepare to close in prayer, suggest that they use the insights about spiritual weapons as they pray. Ask all members to pray silently and encourage all those who feel comfortable doing so to pray aloud.

# Week Five: Prayer: Our Battleground

1. Read John 14:13. Jesus stated He would answer prayer if God's glory were the goal of the prayer. Discuss how we can pray for success in our efforts in the First Place program with the goal of bringing glory

to God. If necessary, follow up with a question about how a change in their lifestyle would bring glory to God. Be sure to mention the changes in prayer life, time spent in Bible study and better eating habits. Remind members that if they can find a solid answer for that question, they can pray with confidence because Jesus has already promised to answer.

2. Spend some time in conversational prayer. Allow volunteers to ask God to use the changes in their lives to bring Him glory.

3. Draw a long horizontal line across the board. At the left end of the line write "faith" and at the right end write "prayer." Above the line write "What's the connection?" Invite members to share their understanding of the connection between prayer and faith. After a few minutes of discussion, have someone read Hebrews 11:6. Discuss what the verse tells them about the connection between faith and prayer. After more discussion, have someone read James 1:6,7. Once again, discuss the connection. Refer to Day 4 for more information.

4. Tell the group they are going to play Point-Counterpoint. Form two groups. Assign Group 1 the responsibility of defending this position: God should have been prepared to answer any prayer asked in faith, not just those that are in line with His will. Assign Group 2 the responsibility of defending this position: We should be glad God only answers prayers that align with His will. Remind each group to defend their assigned position, no matter what they really believe. Give the groups a few minutes to prepare. Allow one group 30 seconds to make a statement defending their position. Allow the other group 30 seconds to respond and 30 more seconds to make another statement. Continue this alternating procedure.

5. Read John 15:7. Explain that God's Word helps us know God's will so that we can pray according to His will. Within God's will we discover the best plan for our lives and the lives of other people.

6. Lead the group in a closing prayer. Thank God for His perfect will and answered prayer.

## Week Six: Motives and Attitudes

1. Ask group members to share what motivated them initially to get involved in the First Place program and lose weight. Instruct them to be as specific and honest as they can.

2. **Before the session**, prepare two large posters. At the top of one poster write "Motives." Draw a vertical line down the center of the poster. On the upper left side of the line write "Negative Motives" and on the upper right side write "Positive Motives." At the top of the second poster write the word "Attitudes." Draw a vertical line down the center; then write "Negative Attitudes" on the upper left side and "Positive Attitudes" on the upper right. Display the posters at this point in the session.

3. Have members form groups of three. Ask each group to evaluate attitudes and motives that help or hinder us in reaching our goals. Ask each group to identify at least three positive and three negative attitudes and three positive and three negative motives. Have them select a spokesperson who will report their insights to the whole group.

4. Bring the whole group back together and have the small groups report. Ask a volunteer to write the groups' insights on the poster. After each group has reported, give everyone an opportunity to ask questions and comment on what was presented.

5. Read Philippians 2:13. Invite volunteers to share how they have seen God increasing their desire to please Him during the past week. Ask others to share how they have sensed God increasing their ability to keep the nine commitments. Remind the group that Philippians 2:13 affirms that God will increase our *want to* and our *can do*.

6. Discuss how thoughts, both positive and negative, impact our attitudes. Read 1 Thessalonians 5:18. Discuss how being thankful can impact our attitudes in a positive way.

7. Lead the group in conversational prayer. Encourage members to pray that God will help them maintain positive attitudes during involvement in the First Place program. Also encourage them to pray that God will help them maintain God-pleasing motives for their goals.

## Week Seven: Run to Win

1. Ask three volunteers to recite Hebrews 12:1 from memory.

2. Invite volunteers to share which box they checked on Day 1. Encourage them to explain their answers.

3. Have members form groups of three. Ask them to share the answers they wrote to the questions on Day 1 about the degree to which their health problems have hindered their Christian lives. Encourage them

to be open and honest so that other members will be able to pray for them and support them in the future.

4. Bring the whole group back together. The apostle Paul often compared the Christian life to an athletic event that required strict training for effective participation. Discuss this concept. Ask how involvement in the First Place program has changed their attitudes about spiritual training.

5. Refer to Day 3. Ask which creates the greatest motivation in their lives: the spiritual prize they can win or the danger of disqualification. Remind the group that Paul used both the positive and the negative to help keep his life on course.

6. Ask someone to read Hebrews 12:1,2. Have the group return to their groups of three and discuss the answer they wrote to the questions (on pp. 101-102) about persevering in the spiritual race.

7. On Day 5, the study focused on finishing the race. In the small groups, ask members to describe the finish line for their goals in the First Place program. Ask them to see themselves crossing the finish line as winners. Have them describe the distance they see between the finish line and where they are right now.

8. Ask members if they have found any other Scripture verses that would help them persevere until they reach their goals. Invite members to share verses and tell how the verses have helped them. Ask if any member can say all seven of the memory verses thus far in the study.

9. Instruct each group of three to close their time of sharing in prayer. Suggest that they pray for one another, asking God to give them strength to persevere in their weight-loss programs until they cross the finish line as winners.

## Week Eight: Handling Temptation

1. Have someone read 1 Corinthians 10:13. Ask volunteers to share some of the strongest temptations they face concerning choices for good health.

2. Give each group member a piece of paper, and instruct members to write out 1 Corinthians 10:13 at the top of the paper. Then give them three minutes to write down as many ideas and insights about facing temptation as possible. After three minutes, ask volunteers to share

one insight or idea. Have one member write the shared ideas on the board or paper.

3.  Instruct everyone to turn to Day 1 and read the four principles drawn from 1 Corinthians 10:13 aloud in unison.

4.  Have members form groups of three. Read 2 Corinthians 10:4,5. Invite members to share their answers to the last three questions for Day 3 with their small groups.

5.  Appoint one person in each group to read James 1:13-15 and 1 John 2:15,16. Instruct the groups to review the material they studied on Day 4 and Day 5; then have them list key insights that can help them understand temptation and how it works in their lives.

6.  Bring the whole group together, and ask one person from each group to report on the insights that they identified. After each group has reported, give an opportunity for comments or questions.

7.  One of the best strategies for overcoming temptation is to avoid it. Discuss practical ways we can avoid the situations that create the temptations.

8.  Ask someone to read J. B. Phillips's translation of 2 Corinthians 12:9,10 (p. 117). Suggest that the group close in prayer by thanking God for the areas of weakness or the strongholds in their lives that provide an opportunity for God to demonstrate His power.

## Week Nine: Handling Guilt

1.  Discuss the ways in which guilt serves the same purpose in our emotional and spiritual lives as fever does in our physical lives.

2.  Ask the group to identify the problem of treating a symptom such as a fever without treating the underlying cause of the fever. Lead them to see that simply telling someone "You don't need to feel guilty about that" may remove a symptom of a deeper spiritual problem without ever dealing with the underlying problem.

3.  Invite volunteers to read Hebrews 10:17 and Psalm 103:12. Discuss the extent to which God has provided a way for us to deal with the underlying cause of guilt in our lives. If necessary, affirm that Christ's death removes our sin and guilt when we become Christians. Through Christ our underlying problem is solved.

4. Have members form groups of three. Refer to Day 4 and discuss the degree to which they could identify with Paul's struggle with sin. Ask if his struggle encouraged or discouraged them and why.

5. Bring the whole group back together. Instruct members to review the material from Day 5. Ask them which idea or insight gained from this study encouraged them the most.

6. Read Galatians 5:25. Discuss how we can keep in step with the Spirit.

7. Revelation 12:10 reveals that Satan is our accuser. Discuss how Satan's accusations can prompt negative feelings of guilt in our lives.

8. Discuss with members their progress in memorizing Scripture. Invite volunteers to share with the group how they have used memorized Scripture in their lives. If no one volunteers, share one of your own experiences using memory verses.

9. Close in prayer, asking volunteers to thank God that in Christ there is no condemnation. After several people have prayed, close the prayer time yourself by praying that each person in your group will experience freedom in Christ—freedom from sin, its strongholds and guilt.

## Week Ten: Knowing God

1. **Before the session**, make seven small posters that list the names of God discussed in this week's study: (1) *Elohim*, the source of all creation; (2) *Jehovah*, the God who is always there; (3) *Jehovah-Jireh*, the God who provides; (4) *Jehovah-Shalom*, the God of peace; (5) *Jehovah-Sabaoth*, God who delivers us; (6) *Jehovah-Rohi*, God our shepherd; (7) *El Roi*, the God who sees.

2. **Before the session**, enlist seven group members who feel comfortable praying aloud. Explain that you will call on them during key times in the session to voice a prayer for the group.

3. Explain that this final session will focus on God, praising Him for who He is and what He has done in their lives during the last 10 weeks.

4. Display the Elohim poster. Review Day 1, and comment on some of the key insights we gain about God and His work through His name, Elohim. Ask one of the seven volunteers to voice a prayer to our powerful God of all creation. Thank Him for the ways He has demonstrated His power to your group during the last 10 weeks.

5.  Display the Jehovah poster. Review Day 2, and comment on the insights members have gained. Have another volunteer voice a prayer to our ever present God, Jehovah. Follow the same procedure with each name of God.

6.  Monitor the time carefully as you lead through each of the names of God. The complete focus on each of the names should take no longer than three minutes.

7.  Ask volunteers to share any strongholds they have been able to overcome this session. Discuss what part the Bible studies, quiet time and prayer played in their victory.

8.  Personally close the session in prayer, thanking God for His work in your life and the lives of others in the group. Thank Him that we have the privilege of knowing and trusting Him. Pray for continued success or effort for the group members.

# How to Fill Out a Commitment Record

The Commitment Record (CR) is an aid for you in keeping track of your accomplishments. Begin a new CR on the morning of the day your class meets. This ensures that your CR is complete before your next meeting. Turn in the CR weekly to your leader.

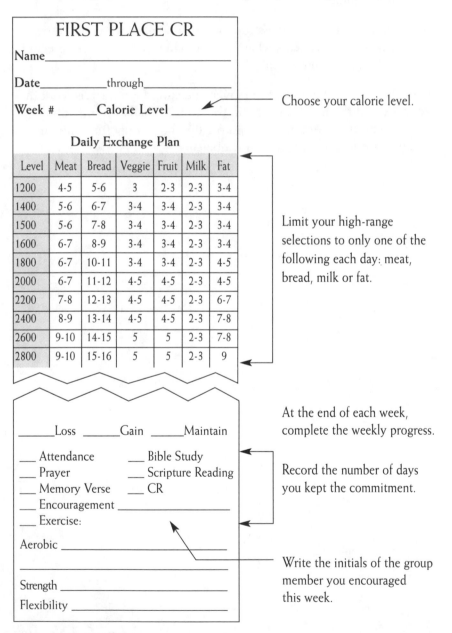

## FIRST PLACE CR

Name_____

Date_____through_____

Week # _____Calorie Level _____

### Daily Exchange Plan

| Level | Meat | Bread | Veggie | Fruit | Milk | Fat |
|-------|------|-------|--------|-------|------|-----|
| 1200 | 4-5 | 5-6 | 3 | 2-3 | 2-3 | 3-4 |
| 1400 | 5-6 | 6-7 | 3-4 | 3-4 | 2-3 | 3-4 |
| 1500 | 5-6 | 7-8 | 3-4 | 3-4 | 2-3 | 3-4 |
| 1600 | 6-7 | 8-9 | 3-4 | 3-4 | 2-3 | 3-4 |
| 1800 | 6-7 | 10-11 | 3-4 | 3-4 | 2-3 | 4-5 |
| 2000 | 6-7 | 11-12 | 4-5 | 4-5 | 2-3 | 4-5 |
| 2200 | 7-8 | 12-13 | 4-5 | 4-5 | 2-3 | 6-7 |
| 2400 | 8-9 | 13-14 | 4-5 | 4-5 | 2-3 | 7-8 |
| 2600 | 9-10 | 14-15 | 5 | 5 | 2-3 | 7-8 |
| 2800 | 9-10 | 15-16 | 5 | 5 | 2-3 | 9 |

_____Loss _____Gain _____Maintain

___ Attendance      ___ Bible Study
___ Prayer          ___ Scripture Reading
___ Memory Verse    ___ CR
___ Encouragement _____
___ Exercise:

Aerobic _____

_____

Strength _____

Flexibility _____

Choose your calorie level.

Limit your high-range selections to only one of the following each day: meat, bread, milk or fat.

At the end of each week, complete the weekly progress.

Record the number of days you kept the commitment.

Write the initials of the group member you encouraged this week.

**DAY 7:** Date _____

Morning _____
_____
_____

Midday _____
_____
_____

Evening _____
_____
_____

Snacks _____
_____
_____

___ Meat _____      ☐ Prayer
___ Bread _____     ☐ Bible Study
___ Vegetable ___     ☐ Scripture Reading
___ Fruit _____     ☐ Memory Verse
___ Milk _____      ☐ Encouragement
___ Fat ___           ☐ Water_____

Exercise:
Aerobic _____
_____
Strength _____
Flexibility _____

List the foods you have eaten. On this condensed CR it is not necessary to exchange each food choice. It will be the responsibility of each member that the tally marks you list below are accurate regarding each food choice. If you are unsure of an exchange, check the Live-It section of your copy of the *Member's Guide*.

List the daily food exchange choices to the left of the food groups.

Use tally marks for the actual food and water consumed.

Check off commitments completed. Use tally marks to record each 8-oz. serving of water.

List type and duration of exercise.

Name _____

Date _____ through _____

Week # _____ Calorie Level _____

## Daily Exchange Plan

| Level | Meat | Bread | Veggie | Fruit | Milk | Fat |
|---|---|---|---|---|---|---|
| 1200 | 4-5 | 5-6 | 3 | 2-3 | 2-3 | 3-4 |
| 1400 | 5-6 | 6-7 | 3-4 | 3-4 | 2-3 | 3-4 |
| 1500 | 5-6 | 7-8 | 3-4 | 3-4 | 2-3 | 3-4 |
| 1600 | 6-7 | 8-9 | 3-4 | 3-4 | 2-3 | 3-4 |
| 1800 | 6-7 | 10-11 | 3-4 | 3-4 | 2-3 | 4-5 |
| 2000 | 6-7 | 11-12 | 4-5 | 4-5 | 2-3 | 4-5 |
| 2200 | 7-8 | 12-13 | 4-5 | 4-5 | 2-3 | 6-7 |
| 2400 | 8-9 | 13-14 | 4-5 | 4-5 | 2-3 | 7-8 |
| 2600 | 9-10 | 14-15 | 5 | 5 | 2-3 | 7-8 |
| 2800 | 9-10 | 15-16 | 5 | 5 | 2-3 | 9 |

You may always choose the high range of vegetables and fruits. Limit your high range selections to only one of the following: meat, bread, milk or fat.

_____ Loss    _____ Gain    _____ Maintain

_____ Attendance    _____ Bible Study
_____ Prayer    _____ Scripture Reading
_____ Memory Verse    _____ CR
_____ Encouragement:
_____ Exercise:
_____ Aerobic
_____ Strength
_____ Flexibility

---

## DAY 7: Date _____

Morning _____

Midday _____

Evening _____

Snacks _____

_____ Meat          ☐ Prayer
_____ Bread         ☐ Bible Study
_____ Vegetable     ☐ Scripture Reading
_____ Fruit         ☐ Memory Verse
_____ Milk          ☐ Encouragement
_____ Fat           ☐ Water

Exercise:
Aerobic _____

Strength _____
Flexibility _____

---

## DAY 6: Date _____

Morning _____

Midday _____

Evening _____

Snacks _____

_____ Meat          ☐ Prayer
_____ Bread         ☐ Bible Study
_____ Vegetable     ☐ Scripture Reading
_____ Fruit         ☐ Memory Verse
_____ Milk          ☐ Encouragement
_____ Fat           ☐ Water

Exercise:
Aerobic _____

Strength _____
Flexibility _____

---

## DAY 5: Date _____

Morning _____

Midday _____

Evening _____

Snacks _____

_____ Meat          ☐ Prayer
_____ Bread         ☐ Bible Study
_____ Vegetable     ☐ Scripture Reading
_____ Fruit         ☐ Memory Verse
_____ Milk          ☐ Encouragement
_____ Fat           ☐ Water

Exercise:
Aerobic _____

Strength _____
Flexibility _____

## DAY 1: Date _____

Morning _____

Midday _____

Evening _____

Snacks _____

| | |
|---|---|
| ___ Meat | ☐ Prayer |
| ___ Bread | ☐ Bible Study |
| ___ Vegetable | ☐ Scripture Reading |
| ___ Fruit | ☐ Memory Verse |
| ___ Milk | ☐ Encouragement |
| ___ Fat | ___ Water |

**Exercise:**
Aerobic _____
Strength _____
Flexibility _____

## DAY 2: Date _____

Morning _____

Midday _____

Evening _____

Snacks _____

| | |
|---|---|
| ___ Meat | ☐ Prayer |
| ___ Bread | ☐ Bible Study |
| ___ Vegetable | ☐ Scripture Reading |
| ___ Fruit | ☐ Memory Verse |
| ___ Milk | ☐ Encouragement |
| ___ Fat | ___ Water |

**Exercise:**
Aerobic _____
Strength _____
Flexibility _____

## DAY 3: Date _____

Morning _____

Midday _____

Evening _____

Snacks _____

| | |
|---|---|
| ___ Meat | ☐ Prayer |
| ___ Bread | ☐ Bible Study |
| ___ Vegetable | ☐ Scripture Reading |
| ___ Fruit | ☐ Memory Verse |
| ___ Milk | ☐ Encouragement |
| ___ Fat | ___ Water |

**Exercise:**
Aerobic _____
Strength _____
Flexibility _____

## DAY 4: Date _____

Morning _____

Midday _____

Evening _____

Snacks _____

| | |
|---|---|
| ___ Meat | ☐ Prayer |
| ___ Bread | ☐ Bible Study |
| ___ Vegetable | ☐ Scripture Reading |
| ___ Fruit | ☐ Memory Verse |
| ___ Milk | ☐ Encouragement |
| ___ Fat | ___ Water |

**Exercise:**
Aerobic _____
Strength _____
Flexibility _____

Name _____

Date _____ through _____

Week # _____ Calorie Level _____

## Daily Exchange Plan

| Level | Meat | Bread | Veggie | Fruit | Milk | Fat |
|---|---|---|---|---|---|---|
| 1200 | 4-5 | 5-6 | 3 | 2-3 | 2-3 | 3-4 |
| 1400 | 5-6 | 6-7 | 3-4 | 3-4 | 2-3 | 3-4 |
| 1500 | 5-6 | 7-8 | 3-4 | 3-4 | 2-3 | 3-4 |
| 1600 | 6-7 | 8-9 | 3-4 | 3-4 | 2-3 | 3-4 |
| 1800 | 6-7 | 10-11 | 3-4 | 3-4 | 2-3 | 4-5 |
| 2000 | 6-7 | 11-12 | 4-5 | 4-5 | 2-3 | 4-5 |
| 2200 | 7-8 | 12-13 | 4-5 | 4-5 | 2-3 | 6-7 |
| 2400 | 8-9 | 13-14 | 4-5 | 4-5 | 2-3 | 7-8 |
| 2600 | 9-10 | 14-15 | 5 | 5 | 2-3 | 7-8 |
| 2800 | 9-10 | 15-16 | 5 | 5 | 2-3 | 9 |

You may always choose the high range of vegetables and fruits. Limit your high range selections to only one of the following: meat, bread, milk or fat.

_____ Loss _____ Gain _____ Maintain

_____ Attendance _____ Bible Study
_____ Prayer _____ Scripture Reading
_____ Memory Verse _____ CR
_____ Encouragement:
_____ Exercise:
Aerobic _____
Strength _____
Flexibility _____

---

## DAY 7: Date _____

Morning _____

Midday _____

Evening _____

Snacks _____

_____ Meat      ☐ Prayer
_____ Bread     ☐ Bible Study
_____ Vegetable ☐ Scripture Reading
_____ Fruit     ☐ Memory Verse
_____ Milk      ☐ Encouragement
_____ Fat       ☐ Water

Exercise:
Aerobic _____
Strength _____
Flexibility _____

---

## DAY 6: Date _____

Morning _____

Midday _____

Evening _____

Snacks _____

_____ Meat      ☐ Prayer
_____ Bread     ☐ Bible Study
_____ Vegetable ☐ Scripture Reading
_____ Fruit     ☐ Memory Verse
_____ Milk      ☐ Encouragement
_____ Fat       ☐ Water

Exercise:
Aerobic _____
Strength _____
Flexibility _____

---

## DAY 5: Date _____

Morning _____

Midday _____

Evening _____

Snacks _____

_____ Meat      ☐ Prayer
_____ Bread     ☐ Bible Study
_____ Vegetable ☐ Scripture Reading
_____ Fruit     ☐ Memory Verse
_____ Milk      ☐ Encouragement
_____ Fat       ☐ Water

Exercise:
Aerobic _____
Strength _____
Flexibility _____

## DAY 1: Date _____

Morning _____

Midday _____

Evening _____

Snacks _____

| Food | Checklist |
|---|---|
| ___ Meat | ☐ Prayer |
| ___ Bread | ☐ Bible Study |
| ___ Vegetable | ☐ Scripture Reading |
| ___ Fruit | ☐ Memory Verse |
| ___ Milk | ☐ Encouragement |
| ___ Fat | ___ Water |

Exercise:
Aerobic _____
Strength _____
Flexibility _____

## DAY 2: Date _____

Morning _____

Midday _____

Evening _____

Snacks _____

| Food | Checklist |
|---|---|
| ___ Meat | ☐ Prayer |
| ___ Bread | ☐ Bible Study |
| ___ Vegetable | ☐ Scripture Reading |
| ___ Fruit | ☐ Memory Verse |
| ___ Milk | ☐ Encouragement |
| ___ Fat | ___ Water |

Exercise:
Aerobic _____
Strength _____
Flexibility _____

## DAY 3: Date _____

Morning _____

Midday _____

Evening _____

Snacks _____

| Food | Checklist |
|---|---|
| ___ Meat | ☐ Prayer |
| ___ Bread | ☐ Bible Study |
| ___ Vegetable | ☐ Scripture Reading |
| ___ Fruit | ☐ Memory Verse |
| ___ Milk | ☐ Encouragement |
| ___ Fat | ___ Water |

Exercise:
Aerobic _____
Strength _____
Flexibility _____

## DAY 4: Date _____

Morning _____

Midday _____

Evening _____

Snacks _____

| Food | Checklist |
|---|---|
| ___ Meat | ☐ Prayer |
| ___ Bread | ☐ Bible Study |
| ___ Vegetable | ☐ Scripture Reading |
| ___ Fruit | ☐ Memory Verse |
| ___ Milk | ☐ Encouragement |
| ___ Fat | ___ Water |

Exercise:
Aerobic _____
Strength _____
Flexibility _____

# FIRST PLACE CR

Name _____

Date _____ through _____

Week # _____ Calorie Level _____

## Daily Exchange Plan

| Level | Meat | Bread | Veggie | Fruit | Milk | Fat |
|---|---|---|---|---|---|---|
| 1200 | 4-5 | 5-6 | 3 | 2-3 | 2-3 | 3-4 |
| 1400 | 5-6 | 6-7 | 3-4 | 3-4 | 2-3 | 3-4 |
| 1500 | 5-6 | 7-8 | 3-4 | 3-4 | 2-3 | 3-4 |
| 1600 | 6-7 | 8-9 | 3-4 | 3-4 | 2-3 | 3-4 |
| 1800 | 6-7 | 10-11 | 3-4 | 3-4 | 2-3 | 4-5 |
| 2000 | 6-7 | 11-12 | 4-5 | 4-5 | 2-3 | 4-5 |
| 2200 | 7-8 | 12-13 | 4-5 | 4-5 | 2-3 | 6-7 |
| 2400 | 8-9 | 13-14 | 4-5 | 4-5 | 2-3 | 7-8 |
| 2600 | 9-10 | 14-15 | 5 | 5 | 2-3 | 7-8 |
| 2800 | 9-10 | 15-16 | 5 | 5 | 2-3 | 9 |

You may always choose the high range of vegetables and fruits. Limit your high range selections to only one of the following: meat, bread, milk or fat.

_____ Loss  _____ Gain  _____ Maintain

_____ Attendance  _____ Bible Study
_____ Prayer  _____ Scripture Reading
_____ Memory Verse  _____ CR
_____ Encouragement:
_____ Exercise:
Aerobic _____

Strength _____
Flexibility _____

---

## DAY 5: Date _____

Morning _____

Midday _____

Evening _____

Snacks _____

_____ Meat
_____ Bread
_____ Vegetable
_____ Fruit
_____ Milk
_____ Fat

☐ Prayer
☐ Bible Study
☐ Scripture Reading
☐ Memory Verse
☐ Encouragement
Water _____

Exercise:
Aerobic _____

Strength _____
Flexibility _____

---

## DAY 6: Date _____

Morning _____

Midday _____

Evening _____

Snacks _____

_____ Meat
_____ Bread
_____ Vegetable
_____ Fruit
_____ Milk
_____ Fat

☐ Prayer
☐ Bible Study
☐ Scripture Reading
☐ Memory Verse
☐ Encouragement
Water _____

Exercise:
Aerobic _____

Strength _____
Flexibility _____

---

## DAY 7: Date _____

Morning _____

Midday _____

Evening _____

Snacks _____

_____ Meat
_____ Bread
_____ Vegetable
_____ Fruit
_____ Milk
_____ Fat

☐ Prayer
☐ Bible Study
☐ Scripture Reading
☐ Memory Verse
☐ Encouragement
Water _____

Exercise:
Aerobic _____

Strength _____
Flexibility _____

# DAY 1: Date ____

Morning ____

Midday ____

Evening ____

Snacks ____

| | ☐ Prayer |
|---|---|
| Meat ____ | ☐ Bible Study |
| Bread ____ | ☐ Scripture Reading |
| Vegetable ____ | ☐ Memory Verse |
| Fruit ____ | ☐ Encouragement |
| Milk ____ | |
| Fat ____ | |
| Water ____ | |

**Exercise:**
Aerobic ____
Strength ____
Flexibility ____

# DAY 2: Date ____

Morning ____

Midday ____

Evening ____

Snacks ____

| | ☐ Prayer |
|---|---|
| Meat ____ | ☐ Bible Study |
| Bread ____ | ☐ Scripture Reading |
| Vegetable ____ | ☐ Memory Verse |
| Fruit ____ | ☐ Encouragement |
| Milk ____ | |
| Fat ____ | |
| Water ____ | |

**Exercise:**
Aerobic ____
Strength ____
Flexibility ____

# DAY 3: Date ____

Morning ____

Midday ____

Evening ____

Snacks ____

| | ☐ Prayer |
|---|---|
| Meat ____ | ☐ Bible Study |
| Bread ____ | ☐ Scripture Reading |
| Vegetable ____ | ☐ Memory Verse |
| Fruit ____ | ☐ Encouragement |
| Milk ____ | |
| Fat ____ | |
| Water ____ | |

**Exercise:**
Aerobic ____
Strength ____
Flexibility ____

# DAY 4: Date ____

Morning ____

Midday ____

Evening ____

Snacks ____

| | ☐ Prayer |
|---|---|
| Meat ____ | ☐ Bible Study |
| Bread ____ | ☐ Scripture Reading |
| Vegetable ____ | ☐ Memory Verse |
| Fruit ____ | ☐ Encouragement |
| Milk ____ | |
| Fat ____ | |
| Water ____ | |

**Exercise:**
Aerobic ____
Strength ____
Flexibility ____

# FIRST PLACE CR

Name _____

Date _____ through _____

Week # _____ Calorie Level _____

## Daily Exchange Plan

| Level | Meat | Bread | Veggie | Fruit | Milk | Fat |
|---|---|---|---|---|---|---|
| 1200 | 4-5 | 5-6 | 3 | 2-3 | 2-3 | 3-4 |
| 1400 | 5-6 | 6-7 | 3-4 | 3-4 | 2-3 | 3-4 |
| 1500 | 5-6 | 7-8 | 3-4 | 3-4 | 2-3 | 3-4 |
| 1600 | 6-7 | 8-9 | 3-4 | 3-4 | 2-3 | 3-4 |
| 1800 | 6-7 | 10-11 | 3-4 | 3-4 | 2-3 | 4-5 |
| 2000 | 6-7 | 11-12 | 4-5 | 4-5 | 2-3 | 4-5 |
| 2200 | 7-8 | 12-13 | 4-5 | 4-5 | 2-3 | 6-7 |
| 2400 | 8-9 | 13-14 | 4-5 | 4-5 | 2-3 | 7-8 |
| 2600 | 9-10 | 14-15 | 5 | 5 | 2-3 | 7-8 |
| 2800 | 9-10 | 15-16 | 5 | 5 | 2-3 | 9 |

You may always choose the high range of vegetables and fruits. Limit your high range selections to only one of the following: meat, bread, milk or fat.

_____ Loss      _____ Gain      _____ Maintain

_____ Attendance       _____ Bible Study
_____ Prayer           _____ Scripture Reading
_____ Memory Verse     _____ CR
_____ Encouragement:
_____ Exercise:
Aerobic _____

Strength _____
Flexibility _____

---

DAY 5:  Date _____

Morning _____

Midday _____

Evening _____

Snacks _____

_____ Meat
_____ Bread
_____ Vegetable
_____ Fruit
_____ Milk
_____ Fat

☐ Prayer
☐ Bible Study
☐ Scripture Reading
☐ Memory Verse
☐ Encouragement
_____ Water

Exercise:
Aerobic _____

Strength _____
Flexibility _____

---

DAY 6:  Date _____

Morning _____

Midday _____

Evening _____

Snacks _____

_____ Meat
_____ Bread
_____ Vegetable
_____ Fruit
_____ Milk
_____ Fat

☐ Prayer
☐ Bible Study
☐ Scripture Reading
☐ Memory Verse
☐ Encouragement
_____ Water

Exercise:
Aerobic _____

Strength _____
Flexibility _____

---

DAY 7:  Date _____

Morning _____

Midday _____

Evening _____

Snacks _____

_____ Meat
_____ Bread
_____ Vegetable
_____ Fruit
_____ Milk
_____ Fat

☐ Prayer
☐ Bible Study
☐ Scripture Reading
☐ Memory Verse
☐ Encouragement
_____ Water

Exercise:
Aerobic _____

Strength _____
Flexibility _____

## DAY 1: Date _____

Morning _____

Midday _____

Evening _____

Snacks _____

| ___ Meat | ☐ Prayer |
| ___ Bread | ☐ Bible Study |
| ___ Vegetable | ☐ Scripture Reading |
| ___ Fruit | ☐ Memory Verse |
| ___ Milk | ☐ Encouragement |
| ___ Fat | ___ Water |

Exercise:
Aerobic _____
Strength _____
Flexibility _____

## DAY 2: Date _____

Morning _____

Midday _____

Evening _____

Snacks _____

| ___ Meat | ☐ Prayer |
| ___ Bread | ☐ Bible Study |
| ___ Vegetable | ☐ Scripture Reading |
| ___ Fruit | ☐ Memory Verse |
| ___ Milk | ☐ Encouragement |
| ___ Fat | ___ Water |

Exercise:
Aerobic _____
Strength _____
Flexibility _____

## DAY 3: Date _____

Morning _____

Midday _____

Evening _____

Snacks _____

| ___ Meat | ☐ Prayer |
| ___ Bread | ☐ Bible Study |
| ___ Vegetable | ☐ Scripture Reading |
| ___ Fruit | ☐ Memory Verse |
| ___ Milk | ☐ Encouragement |
| ___ Fat | ___ Water |

Exercise:
Aerobic _____
Strength _____
Flexibility _____

## DAY 4: Date _____

Morning _____

Midday _____

Evening _____

Snacks _____

| ___ Meat | ☐ Prayer |
| ___ Bread | ☐ Bible Study |
| ___ Vegetable | ☐ Scripture Reading |
| ___ Fruit | ☐ Memory Verse |
| ___ Milk | ☐ Encouragement |
| ___ Fat | ___ Water |

Exercise:
Aerobic _____
Strength _____
Flexibility _____

# FIRST PLACE CR

Name _____

Date _____ through _____

Week # _____ Calorie Level _____

## Daily Exchange Plan

| Level | Meat | Bread | Veggie | Fruit | Milk | Fat |
|---|---|---|---|---|---|---|
| 1200 | 4-5 | 5-6 | 3 | 2-3 | 2-3 | 3-4 |
| 1400 | 5-6 | 6-7 | 3-4 | 3-4 | 2-3 | 3-4 |
| 1500 | 5-6 | 7-8 | 3-4 | 3-4 | 2-3 | 3-4 |
| 1600 | 6-7 | 8-9 | 3-4 | 3-4 | 2-3 | 3-4 |
| 1800 | 6-7 | 10-11 | 3-4 | 3-4 | 2-3 | 4-5 |
| 2000 | 6-7 | 11-12 | 4-5 | 4-5 | 2-3 | 4-5 |
| 2200 | 7-8 | 12-13 | 4-5 | 4-5 | 2-3 | 6-7 |
| 2400 | 8-9 | 13-14 | 4-5 | 4-5 | 2-3 | 7-8 |
| 2600 | 9-10 | 14-15 | 5 | 5 | 2-3 | 7-8 |
| 2800 | 9-10 | 15-16 | 5 | 5 | 2-3 | 9 |

You may always choose the high range of vegetables and fruits. Limit your high range selections to only one of the following: meat, bread, milk or fat.

_____ Loss _____ Gain _____ Maintain

_____ Attendance _____ Bible Study
_____ Prayer _____ Scripture Reading
_____ Memory Verse _____ CR
Encouragement:
Exercise:
Aerobic
Strength
Flexibility

---

## DAY 5: Date _____

Morning _____

Midday _____

Evening _____

Snacks _____

_____ Meat
_____ Bread
_____ Vegetable
_____ Fruit
_____ Milk
_____ Fat

☐ Prayer
☐ Bible Study
☐ Scripture Reading
☐ Memory Verse
☐ Encouragement
Water _____

Exercise:
Aerobic _____

Strength _____
Flexibility _____

---

## DAY 6: Date _____

Morning _____

Midday _____

Evening _____

Snacks _____

_____ Meat
_____ Bread
_____ Vegetable
_____ Fruit
_____ Milk
_____ Fat

☐ Prayer
☐ Bible Study
☐ Scripture Reading
☐ Memory Verse
☐ Encouragement
Water _____

Exercise:
Aerobic _____

Strength _____
Flexibility _____

---

## DAY 7: Date _____

Morning _____

Midday _____

Evening _____

Snacks _____

_____ Meat
_____ Bread
_____ Vegetable
_____ Fruit
_____ Milk
_____ Fat

☐ Prayer
☐ Bible Study
☐ Scripture Reading
☐ Memory Verse
☐ Encouragement
Water _____

Exercise:
Aerobic _____

Strength _____
Flexibility _____

## DAY 1: Date _____

Morning _____

Midday _____

Evening _____

Snacks _____

___ Meat      ☐ Prayer
___ Bread     ☐ Bible Study
___ Vegetable ☐ Scripture Reading
___ Fruit     ☐ Memory Verse
___ Milk      ☐ Encouragement
___ Fat       Water _____

Exercise:
Aerobic _____
Strength _____
Flexibility _____

## DAY 2: Date _____

Morning _____

Midday _____

Evening _____

Snacks _____

___ Meat      ☐ Prayer
___ Bread     ☐ Bible Study
___ Vegetable ☐ Scripture Reading
___ Fruit     ☐ Memory Verse
___ Milk      ☐ Encouragement
___ Fat       Water _____

Exercise:
Aerobic _____
Strength _____
Flexibility _____

## DAY 3: Date _____

Morning _____

Midday _____

Evening _____

Snacks _____

___ Meat      ☐ Prayer
___ Bread     ☐ Bible Study
___ Vegetable ☐ Scripture Reading
___ Fruit     ☐ Memory Verse
___ Milk      ☐ Encouragement
___ Fat       Water _____

Exercise:
Aerobic _____
Strength _____
Flexibility _____

## DAY 4: Date _____

Morning _____

Midday _____

Evening _____

Snacks _____

___ Meat      ☐ Prayer
___ Bread     ☐ Bible Study
___ Vegetable ☐ Scripture Reading
___ Fruit     ☐ Memory Verse
___ Milk      ☐ Encouragement
___ Fat       Water _____

Exercise:
Aerobic _____
Strength _____
Flexibility _____

# FIRST PLACE CR

Name _____

Date _____ through _____

Week # _____ Calorie Level _____

## Daily Exchange Plan

| Level | Meat | Bread | Veggie | Fruit | Milk | Fat |
|-------|------|-------|--------|-------|------|-----|
| 1200 | 4-5 | 5-6 | 3 | 2-3 | 2-3 | 3-4 |
| 1400 | 5-6 | 6-7 | 3-4 | 3-4 | 2-3 | 3-4 |
| 1500 | 5-6 | 7-8 | 3-4 | 3-4 | 2-3 | 3-4 |
| 1600 | 6-7 | 8-9 | 3-4 | 3-4 | 2-3 | 3-4 |
| 1800 | 6-7 | 10-11 | 3-4 | 3-4 | 2-3 | 4-5 |
| 2000 | 6-7 | 11-12 | 4-5 | 4-5 | 2-3 | 4-5 |
| 2200 | 7-8 | 12-13 | 4-5 | 4-5 | 2-3 | 6-7 |
| 2400 | 8-9 | 13-14 | 4-5 | 4-5 | 2-3 | 7-8 |
| 2600 | 9-10 | 14-15 | 5 | 5 | 2-3 | 7-8 |
| 2800 | 9-10 | 15-16 | 5 | 5 | 2-3 | 9 |

You may always choose the high range of vegetables and fruits. Limit your high range selections to only one of the following: meat, bread, milk or fat.

_____ Loss _____ Gain _____ Maintain

_____ Attendance _____ Bible Study
_____ Prayer _____ Scripture Reading
_____ Memory Verse _____ CR
_____ Encouragement:
_____ Exercise:
Aerobic _____
Strength _____
Flexibility _____

---

## DAY 5: Date _____

Morning _____

Midday _____

Evening _____

Snacks _____

_____ Meat
_____ Bread
_____ Vegetable
_____ Fruit
_____ Milk
_____ Fat

☐ Prayer
☐ Bible Study
☐ Scripture Reading
☐ Memory Verse
☐ Encouragement
Water _____

Exercise:
Aerobic _____

Strength _____
Flexibility _____

---

## DAY 6: Date _____

Morning _____

Midday _____

Evening _____

Snacks _____

_____ Meat
_____ Bread
_____ Vegetable
_____ Fruit
_____ Milk
_____ Fat

☐ Prayer
☐ Bible Study
☐ Scripture Reading
☐ Memory Verse
☐ Encouragement
Water _____

Exercise:
Aerobic _____

Strength _____
Flexibility _____

---

## DAY 7: Date _____

Morning _____

Midday _____

Evening _____

Snacks _____

_____ Meat
_____ Bread
_____ Vegetable
_____ Fruit
_____ Milk
_____ Fat

☐ Prayer
☐ Bible Study
☐ Scripture Reading
☐ Memory Verse
☐ Encouragement
Water _____

Exercise:
Aerobic _____

Strength _____
Flexibility _____

## DAY 1: Date _____

Morning _____

Midday _____

Evening _____

Snacks _____

| Food | | Spiritual |
|---|---|---|
| ___ Meat | | ☐ Prayer |
| ___ Bread | | ☐ Bible Study |
| ___ Vegetable | | ☐ Scripture Reading |
| ___ Fruit | | ☐ Memory Verse |
| ___ Milk | | ☐ Encouragement |
| ___ Fat | ___ Water | |

Exercise:

Aerobic _____

Strength _____

Flexibility _____

## DAY 2: Date _____

Morning _____

Midday _____

Evening _____

Snacks _____

| Food | | Spiritual |
|---|---|---|
| ___ Meat | | ☐ Prayer |
| ___ Bread | | ☐ Bible Study |
| ___ Vegetable | | ☐ Scripture Reading |
| ___ Fruit | | ☐ Memory Verse |
| ___ Milk | | ☐ Encouragement |
| ___ Fat | ___ Water | |

Exercise:

Aerobic _____

Strength _____

Flexibility _____

## DAY 3: Date _____

Morning _____

Midday _____

Evening _____

Snacks _____

| Food | | Spiritual |
|---|---|---|
| ___ Meat | | ☐ Prayer |
| ___ Bread | | ☐ Bible Study |
| ___ Vegetable | | ☐ Scripture Reading |
| ___ Fruit | | ☐ Memory Verse |
| ___ Milk | | ☐ Encouragement |
| ___ Fat | ___ Water | |

Exercise:

Aerobic _____

Strength _____

Flexibility _____

## DAY 4: Date _____

Morning _____

Midday _____

Evening _____

Snacks _____

| Food | | Spiritual |
|---|---|---|
| ___ Meat | | ☐ Prayer |
| ___ Bread | | ☐ Bible Study |
| ___ Vegetable | | ☐ Scripture Reading |
| ___ Fruit | | ☐ Memory Verse |
| ___ Milk | | ☐ Encouragement |
| ___ Fat | ___ Water | |

Exercise:

Aerobic _____

Strength _____

Flexibility _____

# FIRST PLACE CR

Name _____

Date _____ through _____

Week # _____ Calorie Level _____

## Daily Exchange Plan

| Level | Meat | Bread | Veggie | Fruit | Milk | Fat |
|---|---|---|---|---|---|---|
| 1200 | 4-5 | 5-6 | 3 | 2-3 | 2-3 | 3-4 |
| 1400 | 5-6 | 6-7 | 3-4 | 3-4 | 2-3 | 3-4 |
| 1500 | 5-6 | 7-8 | 3-4 | 3-4 | 2-3 | 3-4 |
| 1600 | 6-7 | 8-9 | 3-4 | 3-4 | 2-3 | 3-4 |
| 1800 | 6-7 | 10-11 | 3-4 | 3-4 | 2-3 | 4-5 |
| 2000 | 6-7 | 11-12 | 4-5 | 4-5 | 2-3 | 4-5 |
| 2200 | 7-8 | 12-13 | 4-5 | 4-5 | 2-3 | 6-7 |
| 2400 | 8-9 | 13-14 | 4-5 | 4-5 | 2-3 | 7-8 |
| 2600 | 9-10 | 14-15 | 5 | 5 | 2-3 | 7-8 |
| 2800 | 9-10 | 15-16 | 5 | 5 | 2-3 | 9 |

You may always choose the high range of vegetables and fruits. Limit your high range selections to only one of the following: meat, bread, milk or fat.

_____ Loss _____ Gain _____ Maintain

_____ Attendance       _____ Bible Study
_____ Prayer            _____ Scripture Reading
_____ Memory Verse      _____ CR
_____ Encouragement:
_____ Exercise:
Aerobic _____

Strength _____
Flexibility _____

---

## DAY 5: Date _____

Morning _____

Midday _____

Evening _____

Snacks _____

_____ Meat        ☐ Prayer
_____ Bread       ☐ Bible Study
_____ Vegetable   ☐ Scripture Reading
_____ Fruit       ☐ Memory Verse
_____ Milk        ☐ Encouragement
_____ Fat         ☐ Water

Exercise:
Aerobic _____

Strength _____
Flexibility _____

---

## DAY 6: Date _____

Morning _____

Midday _____

Evening _____

Snacks _____

_____ Meat        ☐ Prayer
_____ Bread       ☐ Bible Study
_____ Vegetable   ☐ Scripture Reading
_____ Fruit       ☐ Memory Verse
_____ Milk        ☐ Encouragement
_____ Fat         ☐ Water

Exercise:
Aerobic _____

Strength _____
Flexibility _____

---

## DAY 7: Date _____

Morning _____

Midday _____

Evening _____

Snacks _____

_____ Meat        ☐ Prayer
_____ Bread       ☐ Bible Study
_____ Vegetable   ☐ Scripture Reading
_____ Fruit       ☐ Memory Verse
_____ Milk        ☐ Encouragement
_____ Fat         ☐ Water

Exercise:
Aerobic _____

Strength _____
Flexibility _____

## DAY 1: Date _____

Morning _____

Midday _____

Evening _____

Snacks _____

| | |
|---|---|
| ___ Meat | ☐ Prayer |
| ___ Bread | ☐ Bible Study |
| ___ Vegetable | ☐ Scripture Reading |
| ___ Fruit | ☐ Memory Verse |
| ___ Milk | ☐ Encouragement |
| ___ Fat | ___ Water |

Exercise:
Aerobic _____
Strength _____
Flexibility _____

## DAY 2: Date _____

Morning _____

Midday _____

Evening _____

Snacks _____

| | |
|---|---|
| ___ Meat | ☐ Prayer |
| ___ Bread | ☐ Bible Study |
| ___ Vegetable | ☐ Scripture Reading |
| ___ Fruit | ☐ Memory Verse |
| ___ Milk | ☐ Encouragement |
| ___ Fat | ___ Water |

Exercise:
Aerobic _____
Strength _____
Flexibility _____

## DAY 3: Date _____

Morning _____

Midday _____

Evening _____

Snacks _____

| | |
|---|---|
| ___ Meat | ☐ Prayer |
| ___ Bread | ☐ Bible Study |
| ___ Vegetable | ☐ Scripture Reading |
| ___ Fruit | ☐ Memory Verse |
| ___ Milk | ☐ Encouragement |
| ___ Fat | ___ Water |

Exercise:
Aerobic _____
Strength _____
Flexibility _____

## DAY 4: Date _____

Morning _____

Midday _____

Evening _____

Snacks _____

| | |
|---|---|
| ___ Meat | ☐ Prayer |
| ___ Bread | ☐ Bible Study |
| ___ Vegetable | ☐ Scripture Reading |
| ___ Fruit | ☐ Memory Verse |
| ___ Milk | ☐ Encouragement |
| ___ Fat | ___ Water |

Exercise:
Aerobic _____
Strength _____
Flexibility _____

# FIRST PLACE CR

Name _____

Date _____ through _____

Week # _____ Calorie Level _____

## Daily Exchange Plan

| Level | Meat | Bread | Veggie | Fruit | Milk | Fat |
|-------|------|-------|--------|-------|------|-----|
| 1200 | 4-5 | 5-6 | 3 | 2-3 | 2-3 | 3-4 |
| 1400 | 5-6 | 6-7 | 3-4 | 3-4 | 2-3 | 3-4 |
| 1500 | 5-6 | 7-8 | 3-4 | 3-4 | 2-3 | 3-4 |
| 1600 | 6-7 | 8-9 | 3-4 | 3-4 | 2-3 | 3-4 |
| 1800 | 6-7 | 10-11 | 3-4 | 3-4 | 2-3 | 4-5 |
| 2000 | 6-7 | 11-12 | 4-5 | 4-5 | 2-3 | 4-5 |
| 2200 | 7-8 | 12-13 | 4-5 | 4-5 | 2-3 | 6-7 |
| 2400 | 8-9 | 13-14 | 4-5 | 4-5 | 2-3 | 7-8 |
| 2600 | 9-10 | 14-15 | 5 | 5 | 2-3 | 7-8 |
| 2800 | 9-10 | 15-16 | 5 | 5 | 2-3 | 9 |

You may always choose the high range of vegetables and fruits. Limit your high range selections to only one of the following: meat, bread, milk or fat.

_____ Loss  _____ Gain  _____ Maintain

_____ Attendance  _____ Bible Study
_____ Prayer  _____ Scripture Reading
_____ Memory Verse  _____ CR
_____ Encouragement:
_____ Exercise:
Aerobic

Strength
Flexibility

---

## DAY 7

Morning _____

Midday _____

Evening _____

Snacks _____

| | |
|---|---|
| _____ Meat | ☐ Prayer |
| _____ Bread | ☐ Bible Study |
| _____ Vegetable | ☐ Scripture Reading |
| _____ Fruit | ☐ Memory Verse |
| _____ Milk | ☐ Encouragement |
| _____ Fat | ☐ Water |

Exercise:
Aerobic _____

Strength _____
Flexibility _____

---

## DAY 6

Morning _____

Midday _____

Evening _____

Snacks _____

| | |
|---|---|
| _____ Meat | ☐ Prayer |
| _____ Bread | ☐ Bible Study |
| _____ Vegetable | ☐ Scripture Reading |
| _____ Fruit | ☐ Memory Verse |
| _____ Milk | ☐ Encouragement |
| _____ Fat | ☐ Water |

Exercise:
Aerobic _____

Strength _____
Flexibility _____

---

## DAY 5

Morning _____

Midday _____

Evening _____

Snacks _____

| | |
|---|---|
| _____ Meat | ☐ Prayer |
| _____ Bread | ☐ Bible Study |
| _____ Vegetable | ☐ Scripture Reading |
| _____ Fruit | ☐ Memory Verse |
| _____ Milk | ☐ Encouragement |
| _____ Fat | ☐ Water |

Exercise:
Aerobic _____

Strength _____
Flexibility _____

## DAY 1: Date_____

Morning _____

Midday _____

Evening _____

Snacks _____

____ Meat ____   □ Prayer
____ Bread ____   □ Bible Study
____ Vegetable ____   □ Scripture Reading
____ Fruit ____   □ Memory Verse
____ Milk ____   □ Encouragement
____ Fat ____ ____ Water ____

**Exercise:**
Aerobic _____

Strength _____

Flexibility _____

## DAY 2: Date_____

Morning _____

Midday _____

Evening _____

Snacks _____

____ Meat ____   □ Prayer
____ Bread ____   □ Bible Study
____ Vegetable ____   □ Scripture Reading
____ Fruit ____   □ Memory Verse
____ Milk ____   □ Encouragement
____ Fat ____ ____ Water ____

**Exercise:**
Aerobic _____

Strength _____

Flexibility _____

## DAY 3: Date_____

Morning _____

Midday _____

Evening _____

Snacks _____

____ Meat ____   □ Prayer
____ Bread ____   □ Bible Study
____ Vegetable ____   □ Scripture Reading
____ Fruit ____   □ Memory Verse
____ Milk ____   □ Encouragement
____ Fat ____ ____ Water ____

**Exercise:**
Aerobic _____

Strength _____

Flexibility _____

## DAY 4: Date_____

Morning _____

Midday _____

Evening _____

Snacks _____

____ Meat ____   □ Prayer
____ Bread ____   □ Bible Study
____ Vegetable ____   □ Scripture Reading
____ Fruit ____   □ Memory Verse
____ Milk ____   □ Encouragement
____ Fat ____ ____ Water ____

**Exercise:**
Aerobic _____

Strength _____

Flexibility _____

# FIRST PLACE CR

Name _____

Date _____ through _____

Week # _____ Calorie Level _____

## Daily Exchange Plan

| Level | Meat | Bread | Veggie | Fruit | Milk | Fat |
|---|---|---|---|---|---|---|
| 1200 | 4-5 | 5-6 | 3 | 2-3 | 2-3 | 3-4 |
| 1400 | 5-6 | 6-7 | 3-4 | 3-4 | 2-3 | 3-4 |
| 1500 | 5-6 | 7-8 | 3-4 | 3-4 | 2-3 | 3-4 |
| 1600 | 6-7 | 8-9 | 3-4 | 3-4 | 2-3 | 3-4 |
| 1800 | 6-7 | 10-11 | 3-4 | 3-4 | 2-3 | 4-5 |
| 2000 | 6-7 | 11-12 | 4-5 | 4-5 | 2-3 | 4-5 |
| 2200 | 7-8 | 12-13 | 4-5 | 4-5 | 2-3 | 6-7 |
| 2400 | 8-9 | 13-14 | 4-5 | 4-5 | 2-3 | 7-8 |
| 2600 | 9-10 | 14-15 | 5 | 5 | 2-3 | 7-8 |
| 2800 | 9-10 | 15-16 | 5 | 5 | 2-3 | 9 |

You may always choose the high range of vegetables and fruits. Limit your high range selections to only one of the following: meat, bread, milk or fat.

____ Loss ____ Gain ____ Maintain

____ Attendance ____ Bible Study
____ Prayer ____ Scripture Reading
____ Memory Verse ____ CR
____ Encouragement:
____ Exercise:
Aerobic _____
Strength _____
Flexibility _____

---

## DAY 7: Date _____

Morning _____
_____

Midday _____
_____

Evening _____
_____

Snacks _____
_____

____ Meat    ☐ Prayer
____ Bread    ☐ Bible Study
____ Vegetable    ☐ Scripture Reading
____ Fruit    ☐ Memory Verse
____ Milk    ☐ Encouragement
____ Fat    Water ____

Exercise:
Aerobic _____
Strength _____
Flexibility _____

---

## DAY 6: Date _____

Morning _____
_____

Midday _____
_____

Evening _____
_____

Snacks _____
_____

____ Meat    ☐ Prayer
____ Bread    ☐ Bible Study
____ Vegetable    ☐ Scripture Reading
____ Fruit    ☐ Memory Verse
____ Milk    ☐ Encouragement
____ Fat    Water ____

Exercise:
Aerobic _____
Strength _____
Flexibility _____

---

## DAY 5: Date _____

Morning _____
_____

Midday _____
_____

Evening _____
_____

Snacks _____
_____

____ Meat    ☐ Prayer
____ Bread    ☐ Bible Study
____ Vegetable    ☐ Scripture Reading
____ Fruit    ☐ Memory Verse
____ Milk    ☐ Encouragement
____ Fat    Water ____

Exercise:
Aerobic _____
Strength _____
Flexibility _____

## DAY 1: Date _____

Morning _____

Midday _____

Evening _____

Snacks _____

| | |
|---|---|
| ____ Meat | ☐ Prayer |
| ____ Bread | ☐ Bible Study |
| ____ Vegetable | ☐ Scripture Reading |
| ____ Fruit | ☐ Memory Verse |
| ____ Milk | ☐ Encouragement |
| ____ Fat | ____ Water |

Exercise:
Aerobic _____
Strength _____
Flexibility _____

## DAY 2: Date _____

Morning _____

Midday _____

Evening _____

Snacks _____

| | |
|---|---|
| ____ Meat | ☐ Prayer |
| ____ Bread | ☐ Bible Study |
| ____ Vegetable | ☐ Scripture Reading |
| ____ Fruit | ☐ Memory Verse |
| ____ Milk | ☐ Encouragement |
| ____ Fat | ____ Water |

Exercise:
Aerobic _____
Strength _____
Flexibility _____

## DAY 3: Date _____

Morning _____

Midday _____

Evening _____

Snacks _____

| | |
|---|---|
| ____ Meat | ☐ Prayer |
| ____ Bread | ☐ Bible Study |
| ____ Vegetable | ☐ Scripture Reading |
| ____ Fruit | ☐ Memory Verse |
| ____ Milk | ☐ Encouragement |
| ____ Fat | ____ Water |

Exercise:
Aerobic _____
Strength _____
Flexibility _____

## DAY 4: Date _____

Morning _____

Midday _____

Evening _____

Snacks _____

| | |
|---|---|
| ____ Meat | ☐ Prayer |
| ____ Bread | ☐ Bible Study |
| ____ Vegetable | ☐ Scripture Reading |
| ____ Fruit | ☐ Memory Verse |
| ____ Milk | ☐ Encouragement |
| ____ Fat | ____ Water |

Exercise:
Aerobic _____
Strength _____
Flexibility _____

# FIRST PLACE CR

Name _____

Date _____ through _____

Week # _____ Calorie Level _____

## Daily Exchange Plan

| Level | Meat | Bread | Veggie | Fruit | Milk | Fat |
|---|---|---|---|---|---|---|
| 1200 | 4-5 | 5-6 | 3 | 2-3 | 2-3 | 3-4 |
| 1400 | 5-6 | 6-7 | 3-4 | 3-4 | 2-3 | 3-4 |
| 1500 | 5-6 | 7-8 | 3-4 | 3-4 | 2-3 | 3-4 |
| 1600 | 6-7 | 8-9 | 3-4 | 3-4 | 2-3 | 3-4 |
| 1800 | 6-7 | 10-11 | 3-4 | 3-4 | 2-3 | 4-5 |
| 2000 | 6-7 | 11-12 | 4-5 | 4-5 | 2-3 | 4-5 |
| 2200 | 7-8 | 12-13 | 4-5 | 4-5 | 2-3 | 6-7 |
| 2400 | 8-9 | 13-14 | 4-5 | 4-5 | 2-3 | 7-8 |
| 2600 | 9-10 | 14-15 | 5 | 5 | 2-3 | 7-8 |
| 2800 | 9-10 | 15-16 | 5 | 5 | 2-3 | 9 |

You may always choose the high range of vegetables and fruits. Limit your high range selections to only one of the following: meat, bread, milk or fat.

_____ Loss _____ Gain _____ Maintain

_____ Attendance _____ Bible Study
_____ Prayer _____ Scripture Reading
_____ Memory Verse _____ CR
_____ Encouragement:
_____ Exercise:
Aerobic _____

Strength _____
Flexibility _____

---

DAY 5: Date _____

Morning _____

Midday _____

Evening _____

Snacks _____

_____ Meat      ☐ Prayer
_____ Bread     ☐ Bible Study
_____ Vegetable ☐ Scripture Reading
_____ Fruit     ☐ Memory Verse
_____ Milk      ☐ Encouragement
_____ Fat       ☐ Water

Exercise:
Aerobic _____

Strength _____
Flexibility _____

---

DAY 6: Date _____

Morning _____

Midday _____

Evening _____

Snacks _____

_____ Meat      ☐ Prayer
_____ Bread     ☐ Bible Study
_____ Vegetable ☐ Scripture Reading
_____ Fruit     ☐ Memory Verse
_____ Milk      ☐ Encouragement
_____ Fat       ☐ Water

Exercise:
Aerobic _____

Strength _____
Flexibility _____

---

DAY 7: Date _____

Morning _____

Midday _____

Evening _____

Snacks _____

_____ Meat      ☐ Prayer
_____ Bread     ☐ Bible Study
_____ Vegetable ☐ Scripture Reading
_____ Fruit     ☐ Memory Verse
_____ Milk      ☐ Encouragement
_____ Fat       ☐ Water

Exercise:
Aerobic _____

Strength _____
Flexibility _____

## DAY 1: Date _____

Morning _____

Midday _____

Evening _____

Snacks _____

_____ Meat    _____ Bread    _____ Vegetable    _____ Fruit    _____ Milk    _____ Fat    _____ Water

☐ Prayer    ☐ Bible Study    ☐ Scripture Reading    ☐ Memory Verse    ☐ Encouragement

Exercise:
Aerobic _____
Strength _____
Flexibility _____

## DAY 2: Date _____

Morning _____

Midday _____

Evening _____

Snacks _____

_____ Meat    _____ Bread    _____ Vegetable    _____ Fruit    _____ Milk    _____ Fat    _____ Water

☐ Prayer    ☐ Bible Study    ☐ Scripture Reading    ☐ Memory Verse    ☐ Encouragement

Exercise:
Aerobic _____
Strength _____
Flexibility _____

## DAY 3: Date _____

Morning _____

Midday _____

Evening _____

Snacks _____

_____ Meat    _____ Bread    _____ Vegetable    _____ Fruit    _____ Milk    _____ Fat    _____ Water

☐ Prayer    ☐ Bible Study    ☐ Scripture Reading    ☐ Memory Verse    ☐ Encouragement

Exercise:
Aerobic _____
Strength _____
Flexibility _____

## DAY 4: Date _____

Morning _____

Midday _____

Evening _____

Snacks _____

_____ Meat    _____ Bread    _____ Vegetable    _____ Fruit    _____ Milk    _____ Fat    _____ Water

☐ Prayer    ☐ Bible Study    ☐ Scripture Reading    ☐ Memory Verse    ☐ Encouragement

Exercise:
Aerobic _____
Strength _____
Flexibility _____

# FIRST PLACE CR

Name _____

Date _____ through _____

Week # _____ Calorie Level _____

## Daily Exchange Plan

| Level | Meat | Bread | Veggie | Fruit | Milk | Fat |
|---|---|---|---|---|---|---|
| 1200 | 4-5 | 5-6 | 3 | 2-3 | 2-3 | 3-4 |
| 1400 | 5-6 | 6-7 | 3-4 | 3-4 | 2-3 | 3-4 |
| 1500 | 5-6 | 7-8 | 3-4 | 3-4 | 2-3 | 3-4 |
| 1600 | 6-7 | 8-9 | 3-4 | 3-4 | 2-3 | 3-4 |
| 1800 | 6-7 | 10-11 | 3-4 | 3-4 | 2-3 | 4-5 |
| 2000 | 6-7 | 11-12 | 4-5 | 4-5 | 2-3 | 4-5 |
| 2200 | 7-8 | 12-13 | 4-5 | 4-5 | 2-3 | 6-7 |
| 2400 | 8-9 | 13-14 | 4-5 | 4-5 | 2-3 | 7-8 |
| 2600 | 9-10 | 14-15 | 5 | 5 | 2-3 | 7-8 |
| 2800 | 9-10 | 15-16 | 5 | 5 | 2-3 | 9 |

You may always choose the high range of vegetables and fruits. Limit your high range selections to only one of the following: meat, bread, milk or fat.

___ Loss    ___ Gain    ___ Maintain

___ Attendance       ___ Bible Study
___ Prayer            ___ Scripture Reading
___ Memory Verse      ___ CR
___ Encouragement:
___ Exercise:
Aerobic _____
Strength _____
Flexibility _____

---

## DAY 5: Date _____

Morning _____

Midday _____

Evening _____

Snacks _____

___ Meat          ☐ Prayer
___ Bread         ☐ Bible Study
___ Vegetable     ☐ Scripture Reading
___ Fruit         ☐ Memory Verse
___ Milk          ☐ Encouragement
___ Fat           Water _____

Exercise:
Aerobic _____

Strength _____
Flexibility _____

---

## DAY 6: Date _____

Morning _____

Midday _____

Evening _____

Snacks _____

___ Meat          ☐ Prayer
___ Bread         ☐ Bible Study
___ Vegetable     ☐ Scripture Reading
___ Fruit         ☐ Memory Verse
___ Milk          ☐ Encouragement
___ Fat           Water _____

Exercise:
Aerobic _____

Strength _____
Flexibility _____

---

## DAY 7: Date _____

Morning _____

Midday _____

Evening _____

Snacks _____

___ Meat          ☐ Prayer
___ Bread         ☐ Bible Study
___ Vegetable     ☐ Scripture Reading
___ Fruit         ☐ Memory Verse
___ Milk          ☐ Encouragement
___ Fat           Water _____

Exercise:
Aerobic _____

Strength _____
Flexibility _____

## DAY 1: Date _____

Morning _____

Midday _____

Evening _____

Snacks _____

| ___ Meat | ☐ Prayer |
|----------|----------|
| ___ Bread | ☐ Bible Study |
| ___ Vegetable | ☐ Scripture Reading |
| ___ Fruit | ☐ Memory Verse |
| ___ Milk | ☐ Encouragement |
| ___ Fat | ___ Water |

Exercise:
Aerobic _____
Strength _____
Flexibility _____

## DAY 2: Date _____

Morning _____

Midday _____

Evening _____

Snacks _____

| ___ Meat | ☐ Prayer |
|----------|----------|
| ___ Bread | ☐ Bible Study |
| ___ Vegetable | ☐ Scripture Reading |
| ___ Fruit | ☐ Memory Verse |
| ___ Milk | ☐ Encouragement |
| ___ Fat | ___ Water |

Exercise:
Aerobic _____
Strength _____
Flexibility _____

## DAY 3: Date _____

Morning _____

Midday _____

Evening _____

Snacks _____

| ___ Meat | ☐ Prayer |
|----------|----------|
| ___ Bread | ☐ Bible Study |
| ___ Vegetable | ☐ Scripture Reading |
| ___ Fruit | ☐ Memory Verse |
| ___ Milk | ☐ Encouragement |
| ___ Fat | ___ Water |

Exercise:
Aerobic _____
Strength _____
Flexibility _____

## DAY 4: Date _____

Morning _____

Midday _____

Evening _____

Snacks _____

| ___ Meat | ☐ Prayer |
|----------|----------|
| ___ Bread | ☐ Bible Study |
| ___ Vegetable | ☐ Scripture Reading |
| ___ Fruit | ☐ Memory Verse |
| ___ Milk | ☐ Encouragement |
| ___ Fat | ___ Water |

Exercise:
Aerobic _____
Strength _____
Flexibility _____

# FIRST PLACE CR

Name _____

Date _____ through _____

Week # _____ Calorie Level _____

## Daily Exchange Plan

| Level | Meat | Bread | Veggie | Fruit | Milk | Fat |
|---|---|---|---|---|---|---|
| 1200 | 4-5 | 5-6 | 3 | 2-3 | 2-3 | 3-4 |
| 1400 | 5-6 | 6-7 | 3-4 | 3-4 | 2-3 | 3-4 |
| 1500 | 5-6 | 7-8 | 3-4 | 3-4 | 2-3 | 3-4 |
| 1600 | 6-7 | 8-9 | 3-4 | 3-4 | 2-3 | 3-4 |
| 1800 | 6-7 | 10-11 | 3-4 | 3-4 | 2-3 | 4-5 |
| 2000 | 6-7 | 11-12 | 4-5 | 4-5 | 2-3 | 4-5 |
| 2200 | 7-8 | 12-13 | 4-5 | 4-5 | 2-3 | 6-7 |
| 2400 | 8-9 | 13-14 | 4-5 | 4-5 | 2-3 | 7-8 |
| 2600 | 9-10 | 14-15 | 5 | 5 | 2-3 | 7-8 |
| 2800 | 9-10 | 15-16 | 5 | 5 | 2-3 | 9 |

You may always choose the high range of vegetables and fruits. Limit your high range selections to only one of the following: meat, bread, milk or fat.

_____ Loss _____ Gain _____ Maintain

_____ Attendance _____ Bible Study
_____ Prayer _____ Scripture Reading
_____ Memory Verse _____ CR
_____ Encouragement: _____
_____ Exercise:
Aerobic _____
Strength _____
Flexibility _____

## DAY 5: Date _____

Morning _____

Midday _____

Evening _____

Snacks _____

__ Meat
__ Bread
__ Vegetable
__ Fruit
__ Milk
__ Fat

☐ Prayer
☐ Bible Study
☐ Scripture Reading
☐ Memory Verse
☐ Encouragement
☐ Water

Exercise:
Aerobic _____

Strength _____
Flexibility _____

## DAY 6: Date _____

Morning _____

Midday _____

Evening _____

Snacks _____

__ Meat
__ Bread
__ Vegetable
__ Fruit
__ Milk
__ Fat

☐ Prayer
☐ Bible Study
☐ Scripture Reading
☐ Memory Verse
☐ Encouragement
☐ Water

Exercise:
Aerobic _____

Strength _____
Flexibility _____

## DAY 7: Date _____

Morning _____

Midday _____

Evening _____

Snacks _____

__ Meat
__ Bread
__ Vegetable
__ Fruit
__ Milk
__ Fat

☐ Prayer
☐ Bible Study
☐ Scripture Reading
☐ Memory Verse
☐ Encouragement
☐ Water

Exercise:
Aerobic _____

Strength _____
Flexibility _____

## DAY 1: Date _____    DAY 2: Date _____    DAY 3: Date _____    DAY 4: Date _____

### DAY 1

Morning _____

Midday _____

Evening _____

Snacks _____

| ___ Meat | ☐ Prayer |
| ___ Bread | ☐ Bible Study |
| ___ Vegetable | ☐ Scripture Reading |
| ___ Fruit | ☐ Memory Verse |
| ___ Milk | ☐ Encouragement |
| ___ Fat | ___ Water |

Exercise:
Aerobic _____
Strength _____
Flexibility _____

### DAY 2

Morning _____

Midday _____

Evening _____

Snacks _____

| ___ Meat | ☐ Prayer |
| ___ Bread | ☐ Bible Study |
| ___ Vegetable | ☐ Scripture Reading |
| ___ Fruit | ☐ Memory Verse |
| ___ Milk | ☐ Encouragement |
| ___ Fat | ___ Water |

Exercise:
Aerobic _____
Strength _____
Flexibility _____

### DAY 3

Morning _____

Midday _____

Evening _____

Snacks _____

| ___ Meat | ☐ Prayer |
| ___ Bread | ☐ Bible Study |
| ___ Vegetable | ☐ Scripture Reading |
| ___ Fruit | ☐ Memory Verse |
| ___ Milk | ☐ Encouragement |
| ___ Fat | ___ Water |

Exercise:
Aerobic _____
Strength _____
Flexibility _____

### DAY 4

Morning _____

Midday _____

Evening _____

Snacks _____

| ___ Meat | ☐ Prayer |
| ___ Bread | ☐ Bible Study |
| ___ Vegetable | ☐ Scripture Reading |
| ___ Fruit | ☐ Memory Verse |
| ___ Milk | ☐ Encouragement |
| ___ Fat | ___ Water |

Exercise:
Aerobic _____
Strength _____
Flexibility _____

# FIRST PLACE CR

Name _____

Date _____ through _____

Week # _____   Calorie Level _____

## Daily Exchange Plan

| Level | Meat | Bread | Veggie | Fruit | Milk | Fat |
|---|---|---|---|---|---|---|
| 1200 | 4-5 | 5-6 | 3 | 2-3 | 2-3 | 3-4 |
| 1400 | 5-6 | 6-7 | 3-4 | 3-4 | 2-3 | 3-4 |
| 1500 | 5-6 | 7-8 | 3-4 | 3-4 | 2-3 | 3-4 |
| 1600 | 6-7 | 8-9 | 3-4 | 3-4 | 2-3 | 3-4 |
| 1800 | 6-7 | 10-11 | 3-4 | 3-4 | 2-3 | 4-5 |
| 2000 | 6-7 | 11-12 | 4-5 | 4-5 | 2-3 | 4-5 |
| 2200 | 7-8 | 12-13 | 4-5 | 4-5 | 2-3 | 6-7 |
| 2400 | 8-9 | 13-14 | 4-5 | 4-5 | 2-3 | 7-8 |
| 2600 | 9-10 | 14-15 | 5 | 5 | 2-3 | 7-8 |
| 2800 | 9-10 | 15-16 | 5 | 5 | 2-3 | 9 |

You may always choose the high range of vegetables and fruits. Limit your high range selections to only one of the following: meat, bread, milk or fat.

____ Loss ____ Gain ____ Maintain

____ Attendance ____ Bible Study
____ Prayer ____ Scripture Reading
____ Memory Verse ____ CR
____ Encouragement:
____ Exercise:
____ Aerobic

____ Strength
____ Flexibility

---

## DAY 5: Date _____

Morning _____

Midday _____

Evening _____

Snacks _____

____ Meat          ☐ Prayer
____ Bread         ☐ Bible Study
____ Vegetable     ☐ Scripture Reading
____ Fruit         ☐ Memory Verse
____ Milk          ☐ Encouragement
____ Fat           ☐ Water

Exercise:
Aerobic _____

Strength _____
Flexibility _____

---

## DAY 6: Date _____

Morning _____

Midday _____

Evening _____

Snacks _____

____ Meat          ☐ Prayer
____ Bread         ☐ Bible Study
____ Vegetable     ☐ Scripture Reading
____ Fruit         ☐ Memory Verse
____ Milk          ☐ Encouragement
____ Fat           ☐ Water

Exercise:
Aerobic _____

Strength _____
Flexibility _____

---

## DAY 7: Date _____

Morning _____

Midday _____

Evening _____

Snacks _____

____ Meat          ☐ Prayer
____ Bread         ☐ Bible Study
____ Vegetable     ☐ Scripture Reading
____ Fruit         ☐ Memory Verse
____ Milk          ☐ Encouragement
____ Fat           ☐ Water

Exercise:
Aerobic _____

Strength _____
Flexibility _____

## DAY 1: Date _____

Morning _____

Midday _____

Evening _____

Snacks _____

| ___ Meat | ☐ Prayer |
|---|---|
| ___ Bread | ☐ Bible Study |
| ___ Vegetable | ☐ Scripture Reading |
| ___ Fruit | ☐ Memory Verse |
| ___ Milk | ☐ Encouragement |
| ___ Fat | ___ Water |

Exercise:
Aerobic _____

Strength _____

Flexibility _____

## DAY 2: Date _____

Morning _____

Midday _____

Evening _____

Snacks _____

| ___ Meat | ☐ Prayer |
|---|---|
| ___ Bread | ☐ Bible Study |
| ___ Vegetable | ☐ Scripture Reading |
| ___ Fruit | ☐ Memory Verse |
| ___ Milk | ☐ Encouragement |
| ___ Fat | ___ Water |

Exercise:
Aerobic _____

Strength _____

Flexibility _____

## DAY 3: Date _____

Morning _____

Midday _____

Evening _____

Snacks _____

| ___ Meat | ☐ Prayer |
|---|---|
| ___ Bread | ☐ Bible Study |
| ___ Vegetable | ☐ Scripture Reading |
| ___ Fruit | ☐ Memory Verse |
| ___ Milk | ☐ Encouragement |
| ___ Fat | ___ Water |

Exercise:
Aerobic _____

Strength _____

Flexibility _____

## DAY 4: Date _____

Morning _____

Midday _____

Evening _____

Snacks _____

| ___ Meat | ☐ Prayer |
|---|---|
| ___ Bread | ☐ Bible Study |
| ___ Vegetable | ☐ Scripture Reading |
| ___ Fruit | ☐ Memory Verse |
| ___ Milk | ☐ Encouragement |
| ___ Fat | ___ Water |

Exercise:
Aerobic _____

Strength _____

Flexibility _____

# CONTRIBUTORS

**Jody Wilkinson**, M.D., M.S., the writer of the Wellness Worksheets for this study, is a physician and exercise physiologist at the Cooper Institute in Dallas, Texas. He trained at the University of Texas Health Science Center in San Antonio, Texas, and Baylor University Medical Center in Dallas. Dr. Wilkinson conducts research on physical activity, nutrition and weight management and has worked with the American Heart Association to develop a health program. He believes strongly in using biblical teaching to motivate people to take care of their physical bodies and enjoy abundant living. Jody and his wife, Natalie, have two daughters, Jordan and Sarah, and twin sons, Joel and Cooper.

**Scott Wilson**, C.E.C., A.A.C., the author of the menu plans in this study, has been cooking professionally for 23 years. A certified executive chef with the American Culinary Federation, he currently works in the Greater Atlanta area as a personal chef and food consultant. Along with serving as the national food consultant for First Place, he is a part-time nutrition teacher at Life University and chef/host of a cable cooking show in the Atlanta area, *Cooking 4 Life.* Scott has also authored two cookbooks, *Dining Under the Magnolia* and *Healthy Home Cooking.* In his spare time, he is active in church work and spends time with his wife, Jennifer, and their daughter, Katie.

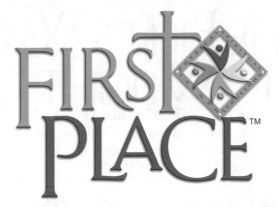

First Place was founded under the providence of God and with the conviction that there is a need for a program which will train the minds, develop the moral character and enrich the spiritual lives of all those who may come within the sphere of its influence.

First Place is dedicated to providing quality information for development of a physical, emotional and spiritual environment leading to a life that honors God in Jesus Christ. As a health-oriented program, First Place will stress the highest excellence and proficiency in instruction with a goal of developing within each participant mastery of all the basics of a lasting healthy lifestyle, so that all may achieve their highest potential in body, mind and spirit. The spiritual development of each participant shall be given high priority so that each may come to the knowledge of Jesus Christ and God's plan and purpose for each life.

First Place offers instruction, encouragement and support to help members experience a more abundant life. Please contact the First Place national office in Houston, Texas at (800) 727-5223 for information on the following resources:

❖ Training Opportunities

❖ Conferences/Rallies

❖ Workshops

❖ Fitness Weeks

Send personal testimonies to:

## First Place

7401 Katy Freeway
Houston, TX 77024

Phone: **(800) 727-5223**
Website: ***www.firstplace.org***

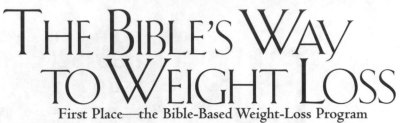
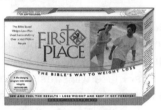

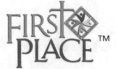

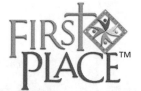

# Available from your local Gospel Light supplier

## First Place Resource Order Form

| TITLE | ISBN/SPCN | QTY | PRICE | ITEM TOTAL |
|---|---|---|---|---|
| First Place Group Starter Kit ($198 Value!) | 08307.28708 | | 149.99 | |
| First Place Member's Kit ($101 Value!) | 08307.28694 | | 79.99 | |
| First Place (Lewis/Whalin) (included in Group Starter Kit) | 00307.28635 | | 18.99 | |
| Choosing to Change (Lewis) (included in Member's and Group Starter Kits) | 08307.28627 | | 8.99 | |
| Giving Christ First Place Bible Study w/Scripture Memory CD (included in Group Starter Kit) | 08307.28643 | | 19.99 | |
| Everyday Victory for Everyday People Bible Study w/Scripture Memory CD | 08307.28651 | | 19.99 | |
| Life That Wins Bible Study w/ Scripture Memory CD | 08307.29240 | | 19.99 | |
| Life Under Control Bible Study w/ Scripture Memory CD | 08307.29305 | | 19.99 | |
| Pressing On to the Prize Bible Study w/ Scripture Memory CD | 08307.29267 | | 19.99 | |
| Seeking God's Best Bible Study w/ Scripture Memory CD | 08307.29259 | | 19.99 | |
| Living the Legacy Bible Study w/ Scripture Memory CD | 08307.29283 | | 19.99 | |
| Pathway to Success Bible Study w/ Scripture Memory CD | 08307.29275 | | 19.99 | |
| Prayer Journal (included in Member's Kit) | 08307.29003 | | 9.99 | |
| Motivational Audiocassettes (pkg. of 4) (included in Member's Kit) | 607135.005988 | | 29.99 | |
| Commitment Records (pkg. o f 13) (included in Member's Kit) | 08307.29011 | | 6.99 | |
| Scripture Memory Verses: Walking in the Word (included in Member's Kit) | 08307.28996 | | 14.99 | |
| Leader's Guide (Included In Group Starter Kit) | 08307.28678 | | 19.99 | |
| Food Exchange Plan Video (included in Group Starter Kit) | 607135.006138 | | 29.99 | |
| Orientation Video (included in Group Starter Kit) | 607135.005940 | | 29.99 | |
| Nine Commitments Video (included in Group Starter Kit) | 607135.005957 | | 39.99 | |
| Giving Christ First Place Scripture Memory Music CD | 607135.005902 | | 9.99 | |
| Giving Christ First Place Scripture Memory Music Cassette | 607135.005919 | | 6.99 | |
| Everyday Victory for Everyday People Scripture Memory Music CD | 607135.005926 | | 9.99 | |
| Everyday Victory for Everyday People Scripture Memory Music Cassette | 607135.005933 | | 6.99 | |
| Life Under Control Scripture Memory Music CD | 607135.006213 | | 9.99 | |
| Life Under Control Scripture Memory Music Cassette | 607135.006206 | | 6.99 | |
| Life That Wins Scripture Memory Music CD | 607135.006237 | | 9.99 | |
| Life That Wins Scripture Memory Music Cassette | 607135.006220 | | 6.99 | |
| Seeking God's Best Scripture Memory Music CD | 607135.006244 | | 9.99 | |
| Seeking God's Best Scripture Memory Music Cassette | 607135.006251 | | 6.99 | |
| Pressing On to the Prize Scripture Memory Music CD | 607135.006268 | | 9.99 | |
| Pressing On to the Prize Scripture Memory Music Cassette | 607135.006275 | | 6.99 | |
| Pathway to Success Scripture Memory Music CD | 607135.006282 | | 9.99 | |
| Pathway to Success Scripture Memory Music Cassette | 607135.006299 | | 6.99 | |
| Living the Legacy Scripture Memory Music CD | 607135.006305 | | 9.99 | |
| Living the Legacy Scripture Memory Music Cassette | 607135.006312 | | 6.99 | |

PRICES SUBJECT TO CHANGE.

11052

**Total : $_____**